Acta Neurochirurgica
Supplements

Editor: H.-J. Reulen
Assistant Editor: H.-J. Steiger

New Trends in Cerebral Aneurysm Management

Edited by
Y. Yonekawa, Y. Sakurai, E. Keller,
and T. Tsukahara

Acta Neurochirurgica
Supplement 82

SpringerWienNewYork

Prof. Dr. Y. Yonekawa
Dr. E. Keller
University Hospital, Zurich, Switzerland

Dr. Y. Sakurai
National Hospital, Sendai, Japan

Dr. T. Tsukahara
National Hospital, Kyoto, Japan

© 2002 Springer-Verlag/Wien

Printed in Austria

Product Liability: The publisher can give no guarantee for all the information contained in this book. This does also refer to information about drug dosage and application thereof. In every individual case the respective user must check its accuracy by consulting other pharmaceutical literature.
The use of registered names, trademarks, etc. in this publication does not imply, even in the absence of specific statement, that such names are exempt from the relevant protective laws and regulations and therefore free for general use.

Typesetting: Asco Typesetters, Hong Kong
Printing: A. Holzhausen, A-1140 Wien
Binding: Fa. Papyrus, A-1100 Wien
Printed on acid-free and chlorine-free bleached paper
SPIN: 10857051

With 63 partly coloured Figures

CIP-data applied for

ISSN 0065-1419
ISBN 3-211-83751-5 Springer-Verlag Wien New York

Preface

The management of cerebral aneurysms is still subject of controversy in spite of recent dramatic advances in surgical techniques and neuro-intensive care. Currently there are three main topics in this field with totally different aspects:

1) management of unruptured cerebral aneurysms as a preventive medicine and
2) neurocritical management of severe subarachnoid hemorrhage (SAH) after rupture and
3) advances in the microsurgical and endovascular techniques regarding the management of cerebral aneurysms.

In order to create an opportunity to discuss these topics, the Swiss-Japanese Joint Conference on Cerebral Aneurysm Management was held in Zurich, Switzerland, from May 5 to 7, 2001; Prof. Dr. Y. Yonekawa, Zurich and Prof. Dr. Y. Sakurai, Sendai were the presidents of the conference. The first day offered a unique forum for European and Japanese neurosurgeons to discuss the treatment of unruptured cerebral aneurysms. In Japan cooperative clinical studies are being carried out on unruptured cerebral aneurysms and presentation of such new clinical experiences allowed intensive discussions in order to find out updated and proper ways to focus the treatment. The second day provided updated information on neurocritical care aspects as well as endovascular and surgical treatment modalities as performed in daily practice in Zurich and Japan. Round table discussions encouraged an interactive communication between the participants and faculty.

In this volume we publish the proceedings of this Swiss-Japanese Joint Conference on Cerebral Aneurysm. Our gratitude is extended to the many contributors and to all those who participated in the conference. Publication of the proceedings is supported by Health Sciences Research Grants for Medical Frontier Strategy Research regarding multi-center studies on the treatment of unruptured cerebral aneurysms by the Japanese Ministry of Health, Labor and Welfare.

The Editors

Contents

Part II: Treatment of Subarachnoid Haemorrhage and General Considerations

Listed in Current Contents

Part I: Management of Unruptured Aneurysms

Acta Neurochir (2002) [Suppl] 82: 3–10

Treatment of Unruptured Cerebral Aneurysms – A Multi-Center Study of Japanese National Hospitals

T. Tsukahara[1], N. Murakami[1], Y. Sakurai[2], M. Yonekura[3], T. Takahashi[4], and T. Inoue[5]

[1] Department of Neurological Surgery and Clinical Research Unit, Kyoto National Hospital, Kyoto, Japan
[2] Department of Neurological Surgery, Sendai National Hospital, Sendai, Japan
[3] Department of Neurological Surgery, National Nagasaki Medical Center, Nagasaki, Japan
[4] Department of Neurological Surgery, Nagoya National Hospital, Nagoya, Japan
[5] Department of Neurological Surgery and Clinical Research Institute, National Kyusyu Medical Center, Fukuoka, Japan

Summary

The treatment and natural course of unruptured cerebral aneurysms were analyzed in 427 cases of unruptured cerebral aneurysm registered at five Japanese national hospitals. Of these cerebral aneurysms 295 were treated by craniotomy, and 22 with endovascular coil embolization. Neurological deterioration after treatment occurred in 31 (9.8%) of the 295 craniotomies and 3 (13.6%) of the 22 endovascular treatments. There was no subarachnoid hemorrhage (SAH) reported after the craniotomies whereas one case of SAH was reported after endovascular treatment. For 145 aneurysms in 110 cases, the natural course of the aneurysms was observed without surgical treatment. During the follow up period of in total 2,610 months (217.5 years), seven of these aneurysms ruptured, resulting in a rupture rate of 3.2%/year. Three of these seven aneurysms were less than 10 mm in diameter. The likelihood of an unruptured cerebral aneurysm to rupture was not exceedingly low. Since the risk of rupture and the morbidity related to surgical treatment cannot be predicted by size alone, the morphology, location and condition of the patients should be considered when treating unruptured cerebral aneurysms.

Keywords: Unruptured cerebral aneurysms; multi center study.

Introduction

Subarachnoid hemorrhage (SAH) due to rupture of a cerebral aneurysm is a serious disorder with a high mortality and morbidity in spite of recent developments in the management of SAH. Therefore it may be reasonable to prevent disastrous SAH and treat cerebral aneurysms before their rupture. With the prevalence of non-invasive methods to detect the cerebral aneurysm, such as MR angiography, we have experienced increasing opportunities to treat patients with asymptomatic unruptured cerebral aneurysms. General consensus for the management of unruptured aneurysms, however, has not yet been established, since there are no prospective randomized trials of treatment intervention versus conservative management. Regarding the natural course of unruptured cerebral aneurysm [3] it is reported that the rupture rate was 10% 10 years after the diagnosis, 26% after 20 years, and 32% after 30 years. Yasui *et al.* reported that the overall rupture rate was 2.3%/year and that the size of these aneurysms was less than 9 mm in 11 of the 22 cases developing SAH. In five cases, aneurysms were even smaller than 5 mm [5, 6]. In 1998, the International Study of Unruptured Intracranial Aneurysms (ISUIA) reported that the rupture rate of cerebral aneurysms smaller than 10 mm was unexpectedly low with 0.05%/year [2]. Although there was criticism that a rather large number of patients with unruptured aneurysms had been excluded from the study after surgeons had indicated a high likelihood of rupture, and only the remaining patients were followed to analyze the natural history [1], this report had rather a big impact on the general public. For example, the Chicago Tribune of December 10, 1998 reported that "A landmark study published Wednesday concludes that brain aneurysms are better left untouched" and "the study found that most small aneurysms won't rupture and attempts to repair them surgically are not worth the risk." Even though these comments did not accurately reflect the contents of the report, treatment indications for unruptured cerebral aneurysms have been markedly influenced by this report. Surgical treatment of unruptured cerebral aneurysm is sometimes unavoidably accompanied by complications, and postoperative results may differ between aneurysms being influenced not only by size but also by localization, morphology and the medical condition of the paient. In 1999, a multi-center study on the treatment of unruptured cerebral aneurysms was organized to accumulate basic data to establish management guidelines for unruptured cerebral aneurysms. The study was supported by a Health Science Research Grant from the Japanese Ministry of Health, Labor and Welfare.

Materials and Methods

Between 1999 and 2000, a total of 427 patients with unruptured cerebral aneurysms were documented in five Japanese national hospitals. Follow-up study of these registered patients is currently going on. For 145 aneurysms in 110 cases the natural course of the aneurysms was observed without surgical treatment. Other cerebral aneurysms were treated surgically either by craniotomy in 295 cases or by endovascular coil embolization in 22 cases. Age distribution of all, surgically treated and untreated patients is shown in Fig. 1a, b and c, respectively. Patients aged 60–69 comprised the peak in each group, although patients of younger age tended to receive surgical treatment while the older group remained untreated. Size of the cerebral aneurysms is shown in Fig. 2a (surgically treated group) and b (untreated group). Aneurysm size was larger in the treated patients. The locations of cerebral aneurysms are shown in Fig. 3a (surgically treated group) and b (untreated group); unruptured cerebral aneurysms were also categorized into four groups by clinical manifestations (Fig. 4a and b): group 1; unruptured cerebral aneurysms accompanied by ruptured aneurysm (23 untreated and 67 treated aneurysms), group 2; unruptured cerebral aneurysms with other intracranial lesions (32 untreated and 97 treated aneurysms), group 3; symptomatic unruptured cerebral aneurysms (12 untreated and 75 treated aneurysms), group 4; incidentally found unruptured cerebral aneurysms (42 untreated and 77 treated aneurysms).

Results

Neurological deterioration occurred after treatment in 31 (9.8%) of 295 craniotomies and 3 (13.6%) of 22 endovascular treatments. There was no SAH reported after the craniotomies and one case of SAH after endovascular treatment. For 145 aneurysms in 110 cases, the natural course of the aneurysms was observed without treatment. During an overall follow-up period of altogether 2,610 months (217.5 years), seven of these aneurysms ruptured, leading to a rupture rate of 3.2%/year. Three of these seven aneurysms were smaller

than 10 mm and two with blebs were even smaller than 5 mm. Four of these seven aneurysms were found incidentally and classified into group IV. The remaining three cases were as follows: two were symptomatic aneurysms (headache and visual disturbance) and one was accompanied by cerebral ischemic disease.

The results of the treatment were analyzed after the aneurysms had been divided according to the age of the patients, size and location of the aneurysms and their clinical manifestations.

Age (Fig. 5a); Outcome of patients at age 80 or more was worse, although the number of surgically treated patients in that age group was small.

Size (Fig. 5b); A greater number of patients with neurological deterioration was reported in patients with an aneurysm larger than 15 mm, although a greater number of neurological improvements was also observed in patients with larger aneurysm.

Location (Fig. 5c); A greater number of patients with neurological deterioration was reported among patients with aneurysms involving the basilar bifurcation compared to those with aneurysms at other sites.

Clinical manifestation (Fig. 5d); In groups I and II, the preoperative medical condition of the patients and accompanying diseases significantly influenced patient outcome. In group III, cranial nerve palsies caused by aneurysms smaller than 10 mm had improved postoperatively in nine cases. However, neurological deficits caused by aneurysms larger than 25 mm had mostly worsened after surgery. In our study, a total of 119 aneurysms were registered as incidental aneurysms in group IV. Aneurysmal size was as follows: 2 to 5 mm in 38 cases, 6 to 9 mm in 42 cases, 10 to 24 mm 32 cases and larger than 25 mm in 3 cases. The percentage of incidentally detected aneurysms measuring less than 10 mm was 67% (80 cases). In one of the 80 cases, aneurysmal size increased over 48 months and clipping of aneurysm was performed. Of 119 incidental cases, 77 cases were treated surgically and 42 cases remained untreated. In four of the 42 untreated cases, the aneurysms had ruptured. In three cases, the size of the aneurysms were larger than 10 mm and the outcome was extremely poor. Two patients died immediately after the rupture and one patient remained in a persistent vegetative state despite surgical treatment. In one patient with three aneurysms measuring less than 5 mm each and with bleb, SAH was reported. Outcome after surgery is shown in Fig. 6. Although the outcome was evaluated by Glasgow outcome scale, 75 of 77 patients showed good recovery, six

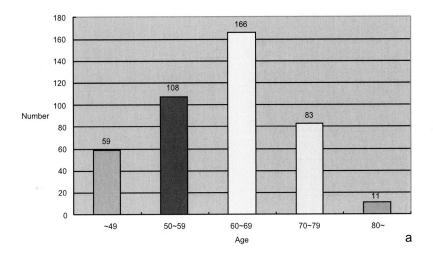

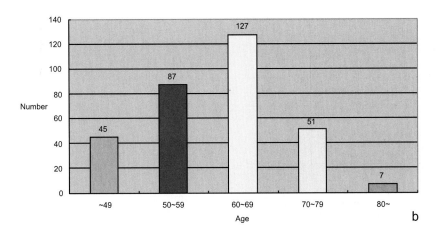

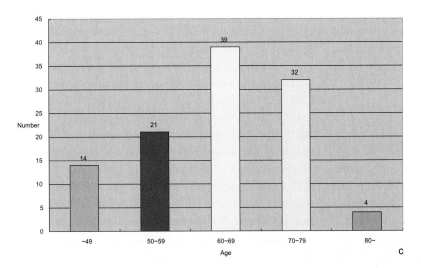

Fig. 1. (a) Ages of all patients with aneurysms. (b) Ages of patients with treated aneurysms. (c) Ages of patients with untreated aneurysms

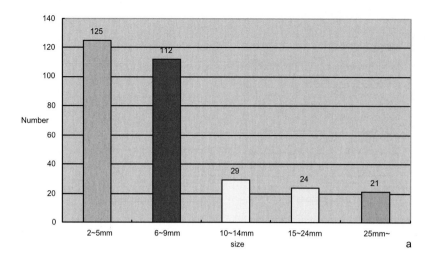

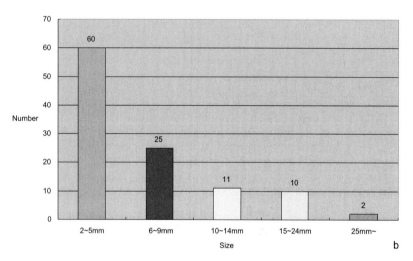

Fig. 2. (a) Sizes of treated aneurysms. (b) Sizes of untreated aneurysms

patients experienced some neurological worsening such as visual field defect after surgery for IC-ophthalmic aneurysm.

Discussion

Decision-making regarding the treatment of unruptured cerebral aneurysms should be based on the natural history and risk of treatment options. At present, however, both the natural course of unruptured cerebral aneurysm and outcome after treatment have not always been clear. Cranial examination using MRI or MR angiography have found asymptomatic cerebral aneurysms in over 2% of total examinees

[4]. These incidental cerebral aneurysms, classified in group IV in our study and detected by brain check-up, differ by nature from symptomatic aneurysms or asymptomatic unruptured aneurysms accompanied by other cerebral lesions. Therefore, management of these aneurysms should be considered separately. In our study, for 145 aneurysms in 110 cases, the natural course of aneurysms was observed without treatment. During the follow-up period of in total 2,610 months (217.5 years), seven of these aneurysms were ruptured resulting in a rupture rate of 3.2%/year. This rupture rate is comparable to previous studies. Four of these seven aneurysms were larger than 10 mm and two of these were fusiform aneurysms of vertebro-basilar arteries. The remaining two were giant aneurysms of

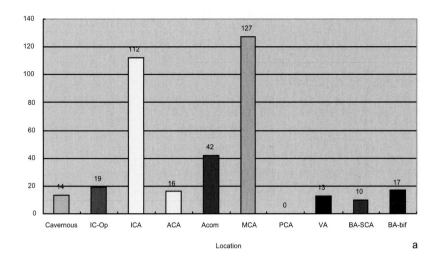

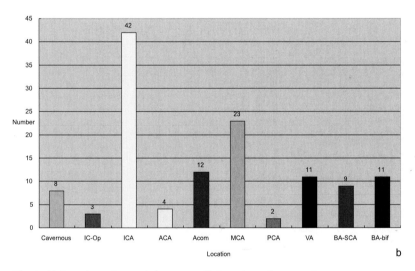

Fig. 3. (a) Locations of treated aneurysms. (b) Locations of untreated aneurysms

IC-ophthalmic and basilar tip. These aneurysms were not treated and observed for their natural course because of the high risk of surgical treatment. The prognosis of these aneurysms is unfortunately rather poor so that we cannot discuss their management at the same time as that of other smaller aneurysms. The main controversy in the management of unruptured cerebral aneurysms is in the management of smaller aneurysms. In our study, three of a total of 85 aneurysms smaller than 10 mm ruptured, and the two with bleb were less than 5 mm. These follow-up results suggested that even smaller aneurysms and aneurysms with bleb could rupture. So although we still cannot identify specific groups at higher risk of cerebral

aneurysm and cannot predict the rupture, small unruptured aneurysms with bleb should be treated surgically if the surgical risk is considered low.

When we estimate the outcome after surgical treatment of unruptured cerebral aneurysm, we have to evaluate not only mortality or morbidity rate but also the quality of life for the patient, including issues related to higher brain function such as cognitive impairment, for example. Since the outcome after treatment varied with the state of the patient before treatment, the results of treatment should be analyzed considering the preoperative neurological status of the patient. In our study, neurological deterioration after treatment of unruptured aneurysms were observed in

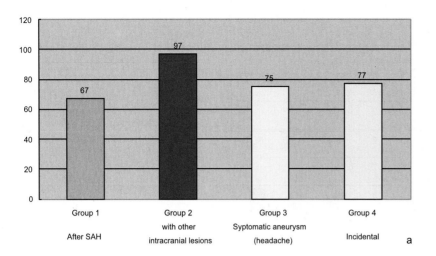

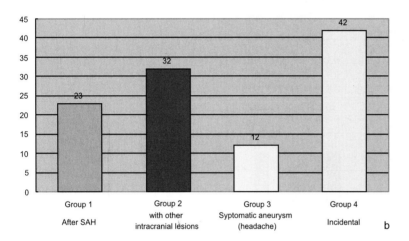

Fig. 4. (a) Conditions leading to diagnosis of the aneurysms. (b) Conditions leading to diagnosis of untreated aneurysms

9.8%; 12% in group I, 7% in group II, 13% in group III and 8% in group IV. These clinical results depend on the preoperative conditions. So in group I or III, the severity of the accompanying diseases, SAH in group I and other neurological disease in group II or III, influenced the outcome of the patient. In group II, five patients died within one year after treatment due to other diseases unrelated to the cerebral aneurysms. Apparently unruptured cerebral aneurysms such as brain tumor or severe systemic diseases are outside the indications for surgery.

In group IV, since patients have no accompanying diseases, the outcome of treatment is better compared with other groups of patients. Seventy five of 77 patients (96.4%) showed good recovery and only 2 cases (2.6%) were mildly disabled when the QOLs of the patients after the treatment were evaluated by the Glasgow outcome scale. However, 8% of patients had some neurological disorder after surgery, we have to develop a new scale to evaluate the surgical results of these patients. In conclusion, since the risk of the rupture and the morbidity related to surgical treatment cannot be predicted by size alone, we must develop a better way to manage unruptured cerebral aneurysms, considering their morphology, location and the condition of the patient.

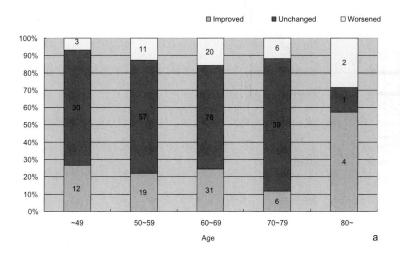

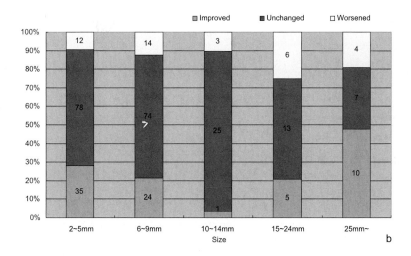

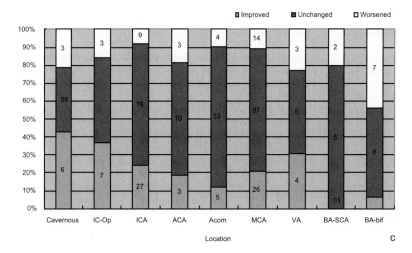

Fig. 5. (a) Surgical outcome with respect to the age of patients. (b) Surgical Outcome with respect to the size of aneurysms. (c) Surgical outcome with respect to the location of aneurysms

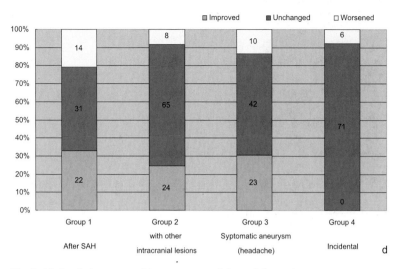

Fig. 5. (d) Surgical outcome with respect to conditions of diagnosis

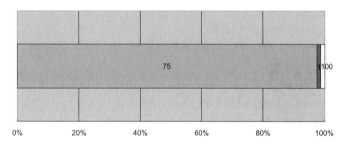

Fig. 6. Surgical outcome of aneurysms discovered incidentally. ■ GR, ■ MD, □ SD, □ PD, ■ D

Acknowledgment

This study is supported by Health Sciences Research Grants from the Japanese Ministry of Health, Labor, and Welfare.

References

1. Ausman JI (1999) The New England Journal of medicine report on unruptured intracranial aneurysms: a critique. Surg Neurol 51: 227–229
2. ISUIA Investigators (1998) Unruptured intracranial aneurysms: risks of rupture and risks of surgical intervention. N Engl J Med 339: 1725–1733
3. Juvela S, Porras M, Heiskanen O (1993) Natural history of unruptured intracranial aneurysms: a long-term follow-up study. J Neurosurg 79: 174–182
4. Nakagawa T, Hashi K (1994) The incidence and treatment of asymptomatic, unruptured cerebral aneurysms. J Neurosurg 80: 217–223
5. Yasui N, Magarisawa S, Suzuki A *et al* (1996) Subarachnoid hemorrhage caused by previously diagnosed, previously unruptured intracranial aneurysms: a retrospective analysis of 25 cases. Neurosurgery 39: 1096–1100
6. Yasui N, Suzuki A, Nishimura H *et al* (1997) Long-term follow-up study of unruptured intracranial aneurysms. Neurosurgery 40: 1155–1159

Correspondence: Tetsuya Tsukahara, M.D., Department of Neurosurgery, Kyoto National Hospital, 1-1 Mukaihata-cho, Fukakusa, Fushimi-ku, Kyoto, 612-8555 Japan.

Acta Neurochir (2002) [Suppl] 82: 11–15

Treatment of Incidental Unruptured Aneurysms

T. Inoue

Department of Neurosurgery, Clinical Research Institute, National Kyushu Medical Center, Fukuoka, Japan

Summary

The most important task for an effective way of SAH prevention is to estimate the rupture risk of unruptured intracranial aneurysms (UIAs) and to reduce the operative risk for clipping. A multi-center study on the treatment of UIAs was organized in 1999, supported by the Japanese Ministry of Health and Welfare. In five Japanese National Hospitals, all UIAs were registered and analyzed.

In this study, we investigated the management outcome in 146 patients with asymptomatic incidentally discovered aneurysms to evaluate the benefit of preventive surgery and conservative treatment. Ninety-seven patients underwent surgery and three patients (3.1%) became moderately or severely disabled after surgery. There was no mortality after surgery or endovascular therapy. Among the 39 patients who underwent conservative therapy, four (10.3%) suffered from subsequent aneurysm rupture. Radical treatment should be considered for the patients with incidental unruptured aneurysms.

Keywords: Incidental unruptured aneurysm; surgery; conservative treatment; subarachnoid hemorrhage.

Introduction

The development of MRA and 3-D CT scan provide a non-invasive method of detecting unruptured intracranial aneurysms (UIAs). However, the indication of radical surgery for UIAs is still obscure [1, 3, 5, 8, 14–17]. Furthermore, the risk of rupture of UIAs has been discussed by several authors, but is still unclear [7, 9–13]. In this article, the results of the Japanese Multi-center study on the treatment of UIAs are presented, in an attempt to elucidate the natural history of unruptured aneurysms and their surgical indication.

Materials and Methods

The records of the patients with a diagnosis of incidental intracranial unruptured aneurysm managed at the departments of neurosurgery in five Japanese national hospitals were reviewed. The multicenter study on the treatment of unruptured intracranial aneurysms was organized on 1999 supported by the Japanese Ministry of Health and Welfare. Unruptured aneurysms were classified into 4 groups: asymptomatic incidentally discovered aneurysms, symptomatic aneurysms, multiple aneurysms in SAH patients, and aneurysms associated with other intracranial disorders. The age, sex, associated medical conditions, clinical presentation, aneurysm size and location were recored for each patient. Outcome was assessed at the last follow-up visit of the patient and categorized according to Glasgow Outcome Scale (GOS). In this study, we investigated the management outcome in 146 patients with asymptomatic incidentally discovered aneurysms.

Results

Patient Characteristics

A summary of the 146 patients with asymptomatic incidentally discovered aneurysms is provided in Table 1. There were 61 men and 85 women. The age at initial diagnosis ranged from 38 to 81 years (mean, 59.2 yr), and 39 to 79 years (mean, 63.5 yr), respectively. Various risk factors for the development of an intracranial aneurysm were documented at the time of diagnosis. There were hypertension in 65 patients (45%), heart disease in 24 patients (16%), diabetes mellitus in 21 (14%), smoking in 20 patients (14%), and polycystic kidney disease in 5 patients (3%). Seven patients (5%) were known to have familial aneurysms.

Table 1. *Summary of 146 Patients with Incidental Unruptured Aneurysm*

Sex	61 (male)	85 (female)	
Ave. of age	59.2 y.o (38–81)	63.5 y.o (39–79)	
Number of aneurysm	116 (single)	29 (multiple)	1 (unknown)
Treatment	97 (surgical)	39 (conservative)	10 (unknown)

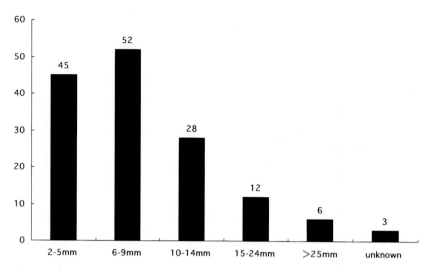

Fig. 1. Size of the largest aneurysm

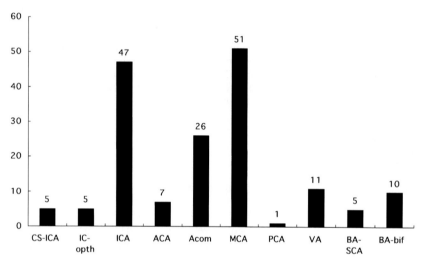

Fig. 2. Location of the unruptured aneurysms

Aneurysm Characteristics

Twenty-nine patients (19.9%) had multiple aneurysms. The size of the largest aneurysms was between 2 and 5 mm in 45 patients (30.8%), between 6 and 9 mm in 52 patients (35.6%), between 10 and 14 mm in 28 patients (19.2%), between 15 and 24 mm in 12 patients (8.2%), and greater than 25 mm in 6 patients (4.1%) (Fig. 1). Data on aneurysm site were available in 146 patients for 168 aneurysms (Fig. 2). The majority (141 aneurysms; 83.9%) were located in the anterior circulation (internal carotid artery, anterior and middle cerebral artery, anterior communicating artery), and fewer (27 patients; 16.1%) were in the posterior circulation (basilar, vertebral, and posterior cerebral arteries).

Treatment

A total of 114 aneurysms were treated in 97 patients. Seventy-eight patients (80.4%) underwent clip ligation of their aneurysms, 10 patients (10.3%) underwent aneurysm wrapping, and 9 patients (9.3%) underwent endovascular interventions. In the surgical group, three patients (3.1%) became moderately or severely disabled after surgery, including 1 dementia and 2 hemiparesis (Table 2). No mortality related to operation or endovascular therapy was observed.

The remaining 39 patients who did not receive surgery were followed up at periods ranging from 1 month to 59 months (average; 18.6 months). Among these patients, one case (2.6%) showed an aneurysm increased in size and 4 patients (10.3%) suffered from

Table 2. *Cause of Poor Outcome after Surgical Treatment*

Case	Age/sex	Location	Size (mm)	Treatment	Post op status	Cause of deterioration	GOS
1	64/F	ACoA	10–14	clipping	dementia	perforator injury	MD
2	64/F	MCA	2–5	clipping	hemiparesis	?	SD
3	67/M	ICA	15–24	clipping	hemiparesis aphasia	ischemia	SD

GOS Glasgow Outcome Scale, *MD* moderate disability, *SD* severe disability.

Table 3. *Aneurysm Rupture During Follow-up*

Case	Age/sex	Location	Size (mm)	Rupture from diagnosis (month)	Treatment	GOS
*1	51/M	ACoA	2–5	31	clipping	GR
2	68/F	ICA	10–14	49	–	D
3	73/F	BA-bif	10–14	48	coil emboliza-tion	V
4	73/F	VA	>25	27	–	D

* Multiple aneurysms (BA-bif, MCA, ACoA), *GOS* Glasgow Outcome Scale, *GR* good recovery, *V* vegetative survival, *D* dead.

subsequent aneurysm rupture (Table 3). The location of bleeding aneurysms was as follows: 1 in the anterior communicating artery, 1 in the internal carotid artery, and 2 in the posterior circulation. There were no significant differences in the risk of rupture according to the location and size of aneurysm. Even a very small aneurysm of less than 3 mm ruptured (Fig. 3). The increase in size of the aneurysm was the significant prediction of rupture (Fig. 4).

Discussion

The natural history of unruptured intracranial aneurysms (UIAs) and the risk factors for rupture are still unclear due to a lack of studies with sufficient patient material and follow-up years [7, 9–13, 18]. Generally, the rate of bleeding in patients with unruptured aneurysms is 1 to 2% annually [5, 15, 17]. In Japan, Yasui *et al.* [18] reported the features of 25 patients with SAH resulting from angiographically verified UIAs who were among 360 patients with conserva-

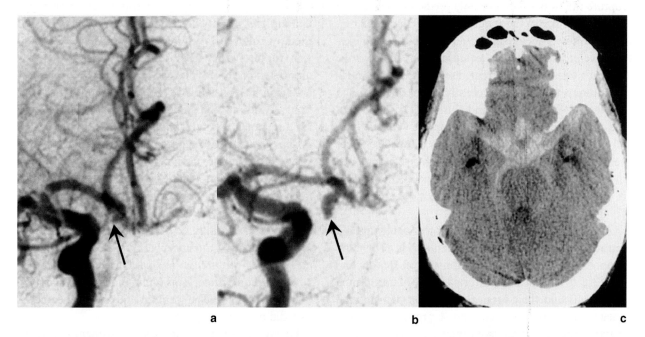

a   b   c

Fig. 3. A 51-year-old man with multiple unruptured intracranial aneurysms (case 1). Right internal carotid arteriogram, on diagnosis (a) and after the rupture (b). The interval increase in size of the anterior communicating artery aneurysm was recognized. (c) CT scan at rupture shows diffuse SAH with interhemispheric hematoma

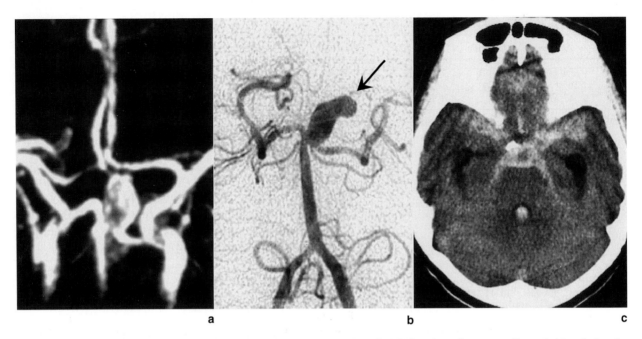

Fig. 4. A 73-year-old woman with unruptured basilar bifurcation aneurysm (case 3). MRA and arteriogram, on diagnosis (a) and after the rupture (b). The interval increase in size of the aneurysm was recognized. (c) CT scan at rupture shows diffuse SAH associated with intra-ventricular hemorrhage of the 4th ventricle

tively treated UIAs. The average annual rupture rate was 2.3% with the risk of rupture of UIAs being higher for multiple aneurysms than single aneurysms. In the study of Juvela et al. Finland [7], the results of 142 patients with 181 UIAs are reported. The average annual rupture rate was 1.4%. The only predictor for the rupture was the size of the aneurysm. They concluded that an unruptured aneurysm should be operated on, irrespective of its size, if it is technically possible and the patient's age and concurrent diseases are not contraindications to surgery. Recently, The International Study of USA, Canada, and Europe [13] stated that the cumulative rate of aneurysm rupture with less than 10 mm in diameter at diagnosis was below 0.05% per year. The surgical treatment of UIAs can only be indicated if the risk of natural history of the disease is higher than the risk of a therapeutic management [2, 4].

A multi-center study on the treatment of unruptured intracranial aneurysms was organized in 1999 and supported by the Japanese Ministry of Health and Welfare, to elucidate the natural history of unruptured aneurysms and their surgical indication. Unruptured aneurysms were classified into 4 groups: asymptomatic incidentally discovered aneurysms, symptomatic aneurysms, multiple aneurysms in SAH patients, and aneurysms associated with other intracranial disorders.

In this study, we investigated the management outcome in 146 patients with asymptomatic incidentally discovered aneurysms. Ninety-seven patients underwent surgery and three patients (3.1%) became moderately or severely disabled after surgery. There was no mortality after surgery or endovascular therapy. Among the 39 patients who underwent conservative therapy, four (10.3%) suffered from subsequent aneurysm rupture. The mean follow-up period was 18.6 months (range, 1–59 m). The aneurysms that ruptured later had increased in size. In the Japanese Hisayama Study, Iwamoto et al. [6] reported that the frequency of ruptured aneurysms was highest in the vertebrobasilar system. But our data suggest that there is no difference between the rupture risk of anterior and posterior circulation aneurysms. One (25%) of 4 aneurysms that later ruptured was 3 mm or less in diameter. Usually, the largest aneurysm is likely to rupture in patients with multiple unruptured aneurysms [7, 13, 15]. However, the smallest aneurysm of 3 mm or less in diameter actually ruptured in one patient who had another two unruptured aneurysms 6 mm or larger in diameter (Table 3. Case 1). The location and size of the aneurysm did not seem to predict rupture.

Our results suggest that radical treatment should be considered for the patients with incidental unruptured aneurysms.

References

1. Asari S, Ohmoto T (1993) Natural history and risk factors of unruptured cerebral aneurysms. Clin Neurol Neurosurg 95: 205–214
2. Ausman J (1999) The New England Journal of Medicine Report on unruptured intracranial aneurysm: a critique. Surg Neurol 51: 227–229
3. Dell S (1982) Asymptomatic cerebral aneurysm: assessment of its risk of rupture. Neurosurgery 10: 162–166
4. Dickey PS, Andreeva L, Kailasnath P (2000) Do selection and referral dias explain the apparent 10 mm rupture threshold for unruptured aneurysms? J Neurosurg 92: 544
5. Heiskanen O (1986) Risks of surgery for unruptured intracranial aneurysms. J Neurosurg 65: 451–453
6. Iwamoto H, Kiyohara Y, Fujishima M (1999) Prevalence of intracranial saccular aneurysms in a Japanese Community based on a consecutive autopsy series during a 30-year observation period. The Hisayama Study. Stroke 30: 1390–1395
7. Juvela S, Porras M, Heiskanen O (1993) Natural history of unruptured intracranial aneurysms: a long-term follow-up study. J Neurosurg 79: 174–182
8. Kassell NF, Torner JC, Haley EC, Jane JA, Adams HP, Kongable GL (1990) The International Cooperative Study on the Timing of Aneurysm Surgery: Part1-Overall management results. J Neurosurg 73: 18–36
9. Khanna RK, Malik GM, Qureshi N (1996) Predicting outcome following surgical treatment of unruptured intracranial aneurysms: a proposed grading system. J Neurosurg 84: 49–54
10. Nakagawa T, Hashi K (1994) The incidence and treatment of asymptomatic, unruptured cerebral aneurysms. J Neurosurg 80: 217–223
11. Raaymakers TW, Rinkel GJ, Limburg M *et al* (1998) Mortality and morbidity of surgery for unruptured intracranial aneurysms: a meta-analysis. Stroke 29: 1531–1538
12. Schievink WI, Piepgras DG, Wirth FP (1992) Rupture of previously documented small asymptomatic saccular intracranial aneurysms: report of three cases. J Neurosurg 76: 1019–1024
13. The International Study of Unruptured Intracranial Aneurysms Investigators: Unruptured intracranial aneurysms-risk of rupture and risks of surgical intervention. N Engl Med 339: 1725–1733, 1998.
14. van Crevel H, Habbema JD, Braakman R (1986) Decision analysis of the management of incidental intracranial saccular aneurysms. Neurology 36: 1335–1339
15. Wiebers DO, Whisnant JP, Sundt TM Jr, O'Fallon WN (1987) The significance of unruptured intracranial saccular aneurysms. J Neurosurg 66: 23–29
16. Winn HR, Almaani WS, Berga SL, Jane JA, Richardson AE (1983) The long-term outcome in patients with multiple aneurysms: incidence of late hemorrhage and implications for treatment of incidental aneurysms. J Neurosurg 59: 642–651
17. Wirth FP, Laws ER Jr, Piepgras D, Scott RM (1983) Surgical treatment of incidental intracranial aneurysms. Neurosurgery 12: 507–511
18. Yasui N, Suzuki A, Nishimura H (1997) Long-term follow-up study of unruptured intracranial aneurysms. Neurosurgery 40: 1155–1160

Correspondence: Tooru Inoue, M.D., Department of Neurosurgery, Clinical Research Institute, National Kyushu Medical Center, 1-8-1 Jigyohama, Chuoh-ku, Fukuoka, 810-8563, Japan.

Acta Neurochir (2002) [Suppl] 82: 17–19

The Treatment of Symptomatic Unruptured Aneurysms

T. Takahashi

Department of Neurosurgery, Nagoya National Hospital, Nagoya, Japan

Summary

The authors analysed 99 cases of symptomatic unruptured aneurysms amongst 427 cases which were collected from a multi-center study of Japanese national hospitals.

There were 20 cases of giant aneurysms and 19 cases of posterior fossa aneurysms. Overall postoperative morbidity was 16%, and postoperative morbidity for giant aneurysms was 26%. The treatment of giant aneurysms and posterior fossa aneurysms proved to be very difficult according to our study.

Keywords: Cerebral aneurysm; non-ruptured; symptomatic; treatment.

Object

We studied the natural course and surgical outcome of unruptured aneurysms, which were collected from a multi-center study of Japanese national hospitals. Among 427 cases of unruptured aneurysms accumulated from the multi-center study, 99 cases of symptomatic aneurysms were analysed. Of the 99 patients, 85 were treated surgically and 14 patients were followed up without surgical treatment. Of the 14 patients followed up conservatively, 2 patients had experienced subarachnoid hemorrhage.

Clinical Materials

Ninety-nine patients (66 females and 33 males, mean age 60 years) with symptomatic unruptured aneurysms were included in this study of which 83 had single and 16 multiple aneurysms. All patients had various symptoms and consequently went to hospital. Headaches were seen in 58 cases; mass effects in 30 cases, ischemic attacks in 5 cases and convulsions in 3 cases.

Regarding aneurysmal size, giant aneurysms above 25 mm were diagnosed in 20 cases, from 15 to 24 mm in 16 cases, from 10 to 14 mm in 8 cases, from 6 to 9 mm in 33 cases and from 2 to 5 mm in 22 cases (Table 1).

Locations were as follows: ICA in 36 cases, MCA in 26 cases, anterior communicating artery aneurysms in 10 cases, IC-ophthalmic aneurysms in 9 cases, VA in 9 cases, basilar top (bifurcation) in 5 cases, basilar-SCA in 5 cases and IC-cavernous aneurysms in 10 cases (Table 2).

Operative methods were: Direct clippings in 54 cases, wrappings in 10 cases, trappings in 4 cases, proximal ligations in 7 cases, coatings in 2 cases and coil embolizations in 8 cases (Table 3).

Table 1.

⟨Aneurysmal size⟩

1) ≫25 mm	20 cases
2) 15∼24 mm	16 cases
3) 10∼14 mm	8 cases
4) 6∼9 mm	33 cases
5) 2∼5 mm	22 cases

Table 2.

⟨Location⟩

1) ICA	36
2) MCA	26
3) AcomA	10
4) IC. ophthal	9
5) VA	9
6) Basilar top	5
7) BA-SCA	5
8) Cavernous ICA	10

Table 3.

⟨Treatment⟩

1) Direct surgery	
Clipping	54
Wrapping	10
Trapping	4
Proximal ligation	7
Coating	2
2) Others	
Bypass	
Coil emboli.	8

Table 4.

Therapy of giant aneurysms (19)		
1) IC-Cavernous.	6	MD (1)
2) IC. Ophthal.	5	MD (2)
3) ICA	5	MD (1)
4) BA. bif.	3	D (2)

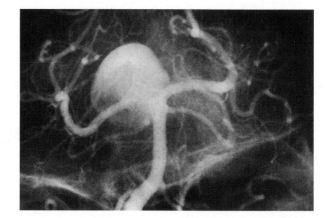

Fig. 1.

Results

Postoperative Results

Postoperative immediate results were as follows. Good recovery in 76 cases, moderate disability in 6 cases, and severe disability in 3 cases. After 3 months, however, postoperative results had deteriorated. 6 cases were worse, 3 were moderately disabled, 2 severely disabled and 3 patients had died. In summary, postoperative morbidity and mortality for symptomatic unruptured aneurysms was 16%.

The treatment of giant aneurysms and posterior fossa aneurysms was very difficult. In our series, 20 cases of giant aneurysms were included:

Six IC cavernous portions, 5 IC ophthalmic, 5 ICA, and 3 basilar bifurcation (Table 4).

For the above method of therapy was 6 direct neck clippings, 4 aneurysmal trappings, 5 ligations and 2 coil embolizations.

Of the 19 giant aneurysms, 5 cases (26%) had a poor outcome.

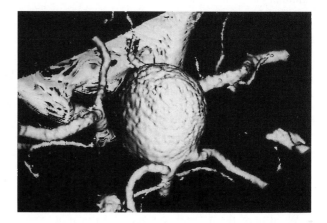

Fig. 2.

Case Presentation

Below we wish to present one of the most difficult cases of giant basilar bifurcation aneurysm: A 56-year-old-man presented at our hospital complaining of throbbing headache. Plain CT showed retrosellar high density mass and the vertebral angiography revealed a giant basilar bifurcation aneurysm protruding antero-superiorly (Fig. 1).

The dome size was 32 mm and the neck width was 9 mm. 3D-CT showed bilateral PCAs and SCAs originating at the posterior aspect of the dome (Fig. 2).

Coil embolization was done by many GDCs with no neurological deficits (Fig. 3).

At the final stage, almost no opacification of the aneurysmal dome was obtained, and main branches were left intact.

Unfortunately, the next morning his systolic blood pressure was suddenly elevated and he complained of headache.

One hour later, he became drowsy and quadriparetic and thereafter became comatose.

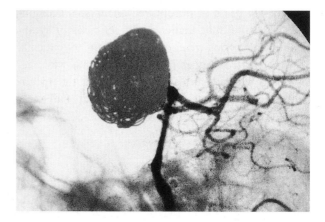

Fig. 3.

An emergently CT scan showed intraventricular hemorrhage and thin subarachnoid hemorrhage.

Two weeks later he died. Complete coil embolization for giant aneurysm was very difficult. The completeness of embolization was not proven even by angiographic control. Coil compaction may be possible in giant aneurysms (Fig. 4).

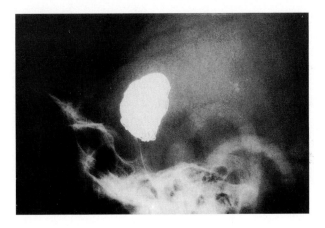

Fig. 4.

Discussion

The treatment of giant aneurysms and posterior fossa aneurysms was very difficult even in unruptured cases [1, 2, 4].

One of the strategy of adequate neck clipping for giant aneurysms was dome shrinkage. Suction and decompression was the chosen method for IC aneurysms and trapping decompression for other aneurysms.

Then the isolation of the neck, many branches and perforators were indispensable [4].

Occasionally, parent artery formation must be done by multiple large ring clips.

The difficulty of basilar bifurcation aneurysmal surgery has well been documented.

Dr. Drake [3], a highly experienced neurosurgeon, reported poor outcome in 12.4% of his operative series.

The causes of poor outcomes he mentioned were perforating artery injury and occlusion of major vessels.

Conclusion

The treatment of symptomatic aneurysms is most difficult, especially in cases of giant aneurysms and basilar bifurcation aneurysms, even by endovascular maneuver.

References

1. Bavinzski G, Killer M, Gruber A *et al* (1999) Treatment of basilar artery bifurcation aneurysms by using Guglielmi detachable coils: a 6-year experience. J Neurosurg 90: 843–852
2. Chyatte D, Porterfield R (2001) Functional outcome after repair of unruptured intracranial aneurysms. J Neurosurg 94: 417–421
3. Drake CG, Peerless SJ, Hernesniemi JA (1996) Surgery of vertebrobasilar aneurysms: London, Ontario experience on 1767 patients. Springer, Wien New York, pp 55–67
4. Tanaka Y, Kobayashi S, Hongo K *et al* (2000) Intentional body clipping of wide-necked basilar artery bifurcation aneurysms. J Neurosurg 93: 169–174

Correspondence: Tatsuo Takahashi, M.D., Department of Neurosurgery, Nagoya National Hospital, 4-1-1, Sanno-maru, Nagoya City, Aichi Prefecture, 460-0001 Japan.

Acta Neurochir (2002) [Suppl] 82: 21–25
© Springer-Verlag 2002

Importance of Prospective Studies for Deciding on a Therapeutic Guideline for Unruptured Cerebral Aneurysm

M. Yonekura

Department of Neurosurgery, National Nagasaki Medical Center, Nagasaki, Japan

Summary

(1) In a town of 100,000 population, a 2% incidence rate of unruptured cerebral aneurysm means 2,000 patients. (2) In a town of 100,000 population, the annual occurrence of subarachnoid hemorrhage is 20. (3) The turnover of patients with unruptured cerebral aneurysm is for the 50-year cycle of patients at age from 30 to 80.

On the basis of these data, in a town of 100,000 population the number of unruptured cerebral aneurysm cases and of subarachnoid hemorrhage cases occurring in 50 years are 2,000 and 1,000, respectively. In total 3,000 patients with unruptured and ruptured cerebral aneurysm, the distribution of these patients for different sizes of aneurysm can be estimated.

We examined the rupture rate for each size of aneurysm. And we found that some of the aneurysm smaller than 10 mm in size rupture soon after their formation and that some of aneurysm of size remain unchanged.

Keywords: Unruptured cerebral aneurysm; rupture rate; growth process of aneurysm; size distribution of aneurysm.

Introduction

An inevitable problem when considering the annual incidence rate of unruptured cerebral aneurysms is whether or not the rate was based on unbiased studies. In 1998, Wiebers *et al.* reported in the New England Journal of Medicine that the annual incidence rate of rupture for unruptured cerebral aneurysms smaller than 10 mm was as low as 0.05% [13]. This value is rather doubtful because it is only 1/20 of the value perceived as normal by most of the neurosurgeons in Japan (1%) [9, 15, 16]. However, data contained in the international study on unruptured intracranial aneurysm must be regarded as reliable owing to an adequate number of aneurysm cases and an adequate period of observation, in spite of a variety of possible biases involved. Up to now, a lot of studies have already been published on patients with subarachnoid hemorrhage and unruptured cerebral aneurysm [2, 5–7, 9, 12, 14]. Based on these data, the author tried to calculate the incidence rate of cerebral aneurysm rupture according to four factors as listed below, and to discuss the importance of prospective studies for determining the guiding principle of treatment for unruptured cerebral aneurysm.

(1) Proportion of patients with unruptured cerebral aneurysm compared to the population concerned.
(2) Proportion of patients with ruptured cerebral aneurysm compared to the population concerned.
(3) Age brackets where cerebral aneurysms occur.
(4) Size distribution of unruptured and ruptured cerebral aneurysms.

Methods, Results and Discussion

First of all, the growth process of cerebral aneurysm from its occurrence may be classified into four patterns, as shown in Fig. 1.

Type 1: The aneurysm ruptures within a time span as short as a few days to a few weeks after its forma-

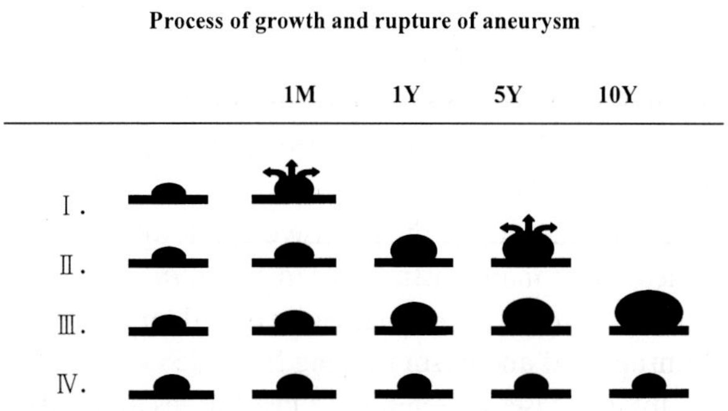

Fig. 1.

Table 1. *Discovery Rate of Cerebral Aneurysm in Autopsy*

		Autopsy	Aneurysm	
1. Riggs & Rupp	(1942)	1,437	131	9%
2. Chason	(1958)	2,786	46	2%
3. Berry	(1961)	6,686	67	1%
4. McCormick	(1965)	2,276	114	5%
5. Inagawa	(1990)	10,259	84	0.8%
Total		21,168	442	2.1%

Table 2. *Discovery Rate of Cerebral Aneurysm in Brain Dock*

'98	A	5567	→	218	(3.9%)
	B	547	→	19	(3.5%)
	C	386	→	19	(4.9%)
	D	1123	→	16	(1.4%)
	E	6189	→	68	(1.1%)
	F	1600	→	44	(2.8%)
'99	G	540	→	9	(1.7%)
	H	1881	→	47	(2.5%)
	I	1639	→	21	(1.3%)
	J	629	→	3	(0.5%)
	K	884	→	92	(10.4%)
'00	L	699	→	41	(5.9%)
	M	880	→	24	(2.7%)
	N	683	→	30	(4.4%)
	O	1646	→	22	(1.3%)
	P	3340	→	57	(1.6%)
	Q	2221	→	97	(4.4%)
	Total	30454	→	825	(2.7%)

Table 3. *Average Annual Subarachnoid Hemorrhage Attack Rates per 100,000 Population*

Poland-Warsaw	10.5	JAPAN	
Sweden-Goteborg	10.5	Shibata	20.0
Denmark-Glostrup	11.0	Jouetsu	16.3
Northern Sweden	17.9	Izumo	21.0
Finland	22.3	Shimane	13.9
USA-Framingham	28.0	Nagasaki	21.0

On the basis of these data, it may be claimed that unruptured cerebral aneurysm exists in about 2% of the total population.

Proportion of Patients with Subarachnoid Hemorrhage Compared to the Population Concerned

There are many reports on the annual incidence rate of subarachnoid hemorrhage resulting from rupture of cerebral aneurysm for a population of 100,000. As shown in Table 3, data in Japan are somewhat different from those in foreign countries: 10 to 28 cases for the overseas and around 20 for Japan.

Age Brackets for Occurrence of Cerebral Aneurysms

The frequency of unruptured cerebral aneurysms and subarachnoid hemorrhage in people younger than 30 is less than 1% of the total population. This means that most of cerebral aneurysms occur in a time span of 50 years from age 30 to 80. In consideration of the three factors mentioned above, the number of patients with unruptured cerebral aneurysm and those with subarachnoid hemorrhage in a town of 100,000 population may be summarized as below.

(A) In a town of 100,000 population, 2% incidence rate of unruptured cerebral aneurysm means 2,000 patients.
(B) In a town of 100,000 population, the annual occurrence of subarachnoid hemorrhage is 20.

For the 50-year cycle of patients with cerebral aneurysm at ages from 30 to 80, the turnover of patients with unruptured cerebral aneurysm may be calculated as

2,000 (persons)/50 (year) = 40 persons/year,

in order to hold the number of unruptured cerebral aneurysms at a fixed level of 2,000 in that town of 100,000 population. That is, in one year, 40 new patients join the symptom group, while 40 succumb to leave the group. The onset of subarachnoid hemor-

tion. Type 2: The aneurysm builds up slowly for a few years after the formation and ruptures in this process. Type 3: The formed aneurysm keeps growing slowly for a few years without rupturing. Type 4: The aneurysm grows up to a certain size, around 10 mm in diameter, and remains unchanged thereafter.

Proportion of Patients with Unruptured Cerebral Aneurysm Compared to the Population Concerned

Autopsy reports in the past indicate that the percent occurrence of unruptured cerebral aneurysm ranged from 0.8% to 9%. Data collected by Riggs [11], Chason, Berry [3], McCormick [10] and Inagawa et al. [4] resulted in 442 sufferings in 21,168 cases (2.1%) (Table 1) [2, 3, 4, 10, 11].

On the other hand, the intensive check-up of brain, carried out in many institutions in Japan these days of patients aged 30 to 70 years, has revealed an incidence of unruptured aneurysm ranging from 0.5% to 10.4%. The total of cases detected in 17 institutions amounted to 825 out of 30,454 cases (2.7%) (Table 2).

Size   Distribution

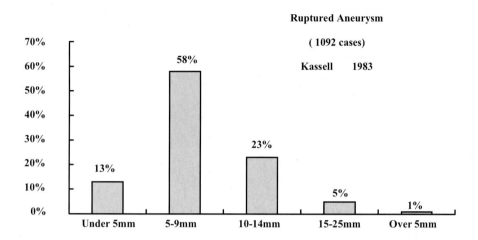

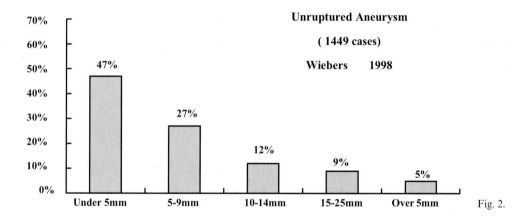

Fig. 2.

rhage amounts to 20 (persons) × 50 (years) = 1,000 persons in 50 years.

Size Distribution of Unruptured and Ruptured Cerebral Aneurysm

In 1983, Kassell *et al.* [8] reported on the size distribution of ruptured cerebral aneurysm based on data from 1,092 cases, while Wiebers *et al.* [13] studied the size distribution of unruptured cerebral aneurysm for 1,449 cases in 1998 (Fig. 2).

Fitting the number of unruptured and ruptured cerebral aneurysm cases calculated according to factors (1), (2) and (3) into the size distribution (4) is shown in Fig. 3.

In a town of 100,000 population, the number of unruptured cerebral aneurysm cases and that of sub-arachnoid hemorrhage cases occurring in 50 years are 2,000 and 1,000, respectively. In total, 3,000 patients with unruptured and ruptured cerebral aneurysms exist, and the distribution of patients for different sizes of aneurysm can be estimated.

Size Distribution in the Town of 100,000 population during 50 years

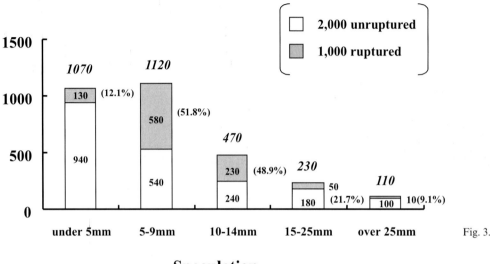

3,000 Aneurysms

Fig. 3.

Speculation

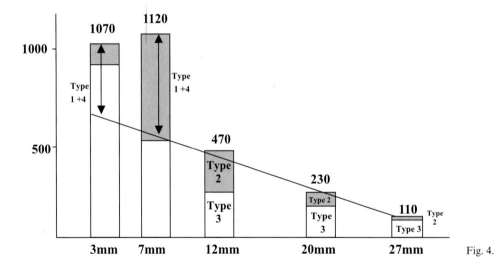

Fig. 4.

In Fig. 4, plots of the number of patients for three size groups of aneurysm, 10–14 mm, 15–25 mm and greater than 25 mm, fall in a straight line of a certain slope, which represents the proportion of patients dying from other disorders while the aneurysm size grows. On the other hand, the number of patients in groups of aneurysm size smaller than 5 mm and 5–9 mm was much greater than that predicted from the growth pattern of types 2 and 3, falling at points above the line. This may suggest that the growth mechanism of aneurysm for this size group involves Types 1 and 4.

It seems, therefore, that the aneurysm of size smaller than 10 mm grows in two different patterns: some rupture immediately after its formation, while the other remain unchanged for a long period. The aneurysm smaller than 5 mm often remains unchanged after its formation. Some of those sized 5–9 mm rupture soon after their formation, and the other of the unruptured group remain unchanged. Looking at Fig. 4 more closely, unruptured aneurysm cases of size 5–9 mm consist of patients with ruptured and unruptured aneurysm sized 10–14 mm, and those unruptured of

10–14 mm size are composed of patients with ruptured and unruptured aneurysm sized 15–25 mm. Finally, patients with unruptured aneurysm of 15–25 mm size include those with ruptured and unruptured aneurysm sized 25 mm or larger.

Conclusion

– Aneurysms larger than 10 mm mostly grow slowly. In patients of this category, the aneurysm ruptures in 48.9% of the 10–14 mm size group, in 21.7% of 15–25 mm, and in 9.1% of 25 mm or larger size.
– Some of the aneurysms smaller than 10 mm in size rupture immediately after formation; the others remain unchanged.

Particularly, aneurysms of a size smaller than 5 mm mostly remain unchanged, while a considerable proportion of 5–9 mm aneurysms rupture immediately after formation.

References

1. Asari S, Ohmoto T (1993) Natural history and risk factors of unruptured cerebral aneurysms. Clin Neurol Neurosurg 95: 205–214
2. Berry RG, Alpers BJ, White JC (1961) The site, structure and frequency of intracranial aneurysms, angiomas and arteriovenous abnormalities. Res Publ Assoc Res Nerv Ment Dis 41: 40–72
3. Chason JL, Hindman WM (1958) Berry aneurysms of the circle of Willis. Results of a planned autopsy study. Neurology 8: 41–44
4. Inagawa T, Hirano A (1990) Autopsy Study of unruptured incidental aneurysms. Surg Neurol 34: 361–365
5. Ingall T, Asplund K, Mähönen M, Bonita R (2000) A multinational comparison of subarachnoid hemorrhage epidemiology in the WHO MONICA Stroke Study. Stroke 31: 1054–1061
6. Juvela S, Porras M, Heiskanen O (1993) Natural history of unruptured intracranial aneurysms: long-term follow-up study. J Neurosurg 79: 174–182
7. Juvela S, Porras M, Poussa K (2000) Natural history of unruptured intracranial aneurysms: probability of and risk factors for aneurysm rupture. J Neurosurg 93: 379–387
8. Kassell NF, Torner JC (1983) Size of intracranial aneurysms. Neurosurgery 12: 291–297
9. Locksley HB (1966) Report on the Cooperative Study of intracranial aneurysms and subarachnoid hemorrhage. Based on 6368 cases in the Cooperative Study. JNS 25: 321–368
10. McCormick WF, Nofzinger JD (1965) Saccular intracranial aneurysms. An autopsy study. J Neurosurg 22: 155–159
11. Riggs HE, Rupp C (1943) Miliary aneurysms. Relation of anomalies of the circle of Willis to formation of aneurysms. Arch Neurol Psychiatry 49: 615–616
12. Wiebers DO, Whisnant JP, O'Fallon WM (1981) The natural history of unruptured intracranial aneurysms. N Engl J Med 304: 696–698
13. Wiebers DO (1998) Unruptured Intracranial Aneurysms – Risk of Rupture and Risks of Surgical Intervention. N Eng J Med 339(24): 1725–1733
14. Yasui N, Magarisawa S, Suzuki A, Nishimura H, Okudera T, Abe T (1996) Subarachnoid hemorrhage caused by previously diagnosed, previously unruptured intracranial aneurysms: a retrospective analysis of 25 cases. Neurosurg 39: 1096–1101
15. Yasui N, Suzuki A, Nishimura H, Suzuki K, Abe T (1997) Long-term follow-up study of unruptured intracranial aneurysms. Neurosurg 40: 1155–1160
16. Yoshimoto T, Mizoi K (1997) Importance of management of unruptured cerebral aneurysms. Surg Neurol 47: 522–526

Correspondence: M. Yonekura, Department of Neurosurgery, National Nagasaki Medical Center, 2-1001-1 Kubara Omura City, Nagasaki, 856-8562 Japan.

Acta Neurochir (2002) [Suppl] 82: 27–30

Natural History of Unruptured Intracranial Aneurysms: Risks for Aneurysm Formation, Growth, and Rupture

S. Juvela

Department of Neurosurgery, Helsinki University Central Hospital, Helsinki, Finland

Summary

Several studies concerning risk factors for SAH and for subsequent rupture of an unruptured aneurysm have been published, but not risk factor studies for formation and growth rate of aneurysms. Because less than half of all aneurysms ever rupture, it is essential to know risk factors separately both for aneurysm formation and for its growth. Before 1979, unruptured aneurysms were not operated on in Helsinki. Recently, the results of risk factors for rupture of unruptured aneurysms of 142 patients (131 with a prior SAH) have been published. 89 were followed with conventional and/or 3D CT angiography, or at autopsy to define risk factors for aneurysm formation and growth. During 2575 person-years, 33 of the 142 patients (23%) suffered SAH, resulting in an annual incidence of 1.3% (95% CI, 0.9–1.7%). The cumulative rate of bleeding was 10.5% (95% CI, 5.3–15.8%) at 10 years, and 30.3% (21.1–39.6%) at 30 years. Independent risk factors for rupture were cigarette smoking (time-dependent relative risk, 3.04; 95% CI, 1.21–7.66), and size of aneurysm (1.14 per mm; 1.01–1.30) after adjustment for age, aneurysm group, and hypertension. In addition, current cigarette smoking at end of follow-up (age-adjusted odds ratio, 3.92; 95% CI, 1.29–11.93) and female gender 3.36 (1.11–10.22) were the only independent risk factors for aneurysm growth of ≥ 1 mm but only current smoking (3.48, 1.14–10.64) was a risk factor for growth of ≥ 3 mm. Probability of de novo aneurysm formation was 0.84% per year (95% CI, 0.47–1.37%). Female gender (adjusted odds ratio, 4.73; 95% CI, 1.16–19.38) and current smoking (4.07, 1.09–15.15) were the only significant ($p < 0.05$) independent risk factors for de novo aneurysm formation. Cessation of smoking is very important for these patients. It is recommended that unruptured aneurysms be operated on irrespective of their size and of patients' smoking status, in people aged <50 to 60 years.

Keywords: Cerebral aneurysm; subarachnoid hemorrhage; cigarette smoking; female gender.

Introduction

The prognosis for aneurysmal subarachnoid hemorrhage (SAH), despite improvements in medical and neurosurgical treatment, has remained largely un-

Table 1. *Risk of Rupture of Unruptured Intracranial Aneurysm*

Study	No. pats	No. SAHs	F-u yrs	Incid./yr	Risk factors
Juvela -00	142	33	2575	1.3	1,3,6
ISUIA -98	1449	32	12023	0.3	1,3,4,7
Yasui -97	234	34	1464	2.3	5
Juvela -93	142	27	1944	1.4	3
Wiebers 87	130	15	1079	1.4	3
Winn -83	38	3/6	380	1.0/2.2	2

1 Age, *2* hypertension, *3* an. diam., *4* an. locat. *5* no. aneurysms, *6* smoking, *7* aneurysm group.

affected [1, 5]. SAH is also the most common form of stroke and cause of stroke mortality among young adults.

During the last few decades, several studies concerning risk factors for SAH (i.e. for ruptured intracranial aneurysm) [1, 5] and for future rupture of a verified unruptured aneurysm (Table 1) [2, 3, 6–9], have been published but not risk factor studies for formation and growth rate of intracranial aneurysms. Because less than half of all aneurysms ever rupture, it is also essential to know risk factors separately both for aneurysm formation and for its growth.

Before 1979, unruptured aneurysms were not operated on in our clinic. Recently, the final results of risk factors for rupture of unruptured aneurysms of 142 patients has been published [3]. In addition, 89 patients of them were followed by conventional angiography and/or by three-dimensional computed tomographic (3D-CT) angiography, or examined at autopsy to define risk factors for aneurysm formation and growth [4].

Table 2. *Multivariate Relative Risks (95% Confidence Intervals) of Cigarette Smoking, Age, and Size of Unruptured Aneurysm for Subarachnoid Hemorrhage*

Characteristic	Model 1	Model 2
Current smoking	1.46 (1.04–2.06)*	3.04 (1.21–7.66)*
Diameter of unruptured aneurysm (per mm)*	1.15 (1.01–1.31)*	1.14 (1.01–1.30)*
Age (per year)	0.97 (0.92–1.01)	0.97 (0.92–1.01)

Relative risks adjusted for the other variables and additionally also for aneurysm group (prior SAH group vs others), sex, and hypertension. In model 1, current smoking is a fixed covariate; in model 2, current smoking is a time-dependent covariate.
* $p < 0.05$.

Material and Methods

For detailed baseline characteristics of the 142 patients (131 with a prior SAH) who were at the Department of Neurosurgery, Helsinki University Hospital, between 1956 and 1978, for aneurysm evaluation as well as inclusion and exclusion criteria of the study, see previous reports [2, 3]. Patients with symptomatic aneurysms were included in the study only if SAH was excluded by a lumbar puncture within a few days after onset of symptoms.

The aneurysm formation and growth part of the study comprised 94 patients, of whom 89 were also included in the study of 142 patients with unruptured aneurysms [3, 4]. Unruptured aneurysms of these patients were later measured either with conventional and/or 3D-CT angiography or at autopsy. In addition, formation of new aneurysms was also registered.

Results

During the follow-up of 2.575 person-years, 33 of the 142 patients (23%) suffered SAH, an approximate annual incidence of 1.3% (95% confidence interval, 0.9% to 1.7%), with an average annual incidence of SAH by group of 2.6%, 1.0% and 1.3% for symptomatic, incidental and prior SAH aneurysm groups, respectively [3]. The 34th patient (non-smoking woman aged 71.8 years) suffered a severe SAH after a follow-up of 23.7 years in February 2000 from an unruptured anterior communicating artery aneurysm of 4 mm in diameter diagnosed in 1976, and which aneurysm was similar on CT angiography performed in 1997. This aneurysm had grown after 1997 and ruptured for the first time in 2000.

The cumulative rate of bleeding in the whole patient population was 10.5% (95% CI, 5.3 to 15.8%) at 10 years after diagnosis of unruptured aneurysm, 23.0% (15.4 to 30.5%) at 20 years, and 30.3% (21.1 to 39.6%) at 30 years [3].

Adjusted multivariate relative risks of significant risk factors for future rupture of unruptured aneurysms are shown in Table 2.

Table 3. *Age-Adjusted Multivariate Odds Ratios (95% Confidence Intervals) of Occurrence of Growth of Unruptured Intracranial Aneurysm*

Characteristic	Patients with angiographic follow-up	All patients
Aneurysm growth, ≥1 mm		
Female gender	3.51 (1.09–11.24)*	3.36 (1.11–10.22)*
Cigarette smoking		
– Quitters	1.20 (0.19–7.69)	1.08 (0.17–6.73)
– Current smokers	3.94 (1.26–12.34)*	3.92 (1.29–11.93)*
Aneurysm growth, ≥3 mm		
Female gender	2.06 (0.64–6.62)	1.91 (0.64–5.68)
Cigarette smoking		
– Quitters	1.77 (0.26–11.91)	1.48 (0.23–9.52)
– Current smokers	3.62 (1.12–11.70)*	3.48 (1.14–10.64)*

* $p < 0.05$.

The largest aneurysm in patients with a follow-up of aneurysm size (n = 87) grew significantly ($p < 0.01$) during the follow-up (mean $\pm$ SD, 2.5 ± 3.7 mm, range 0 to 17 mm; 0.31 ± 0.86 mm/yr; and 12.1 ± 42.5%/yr).

Aneurysms that later ruptured had increased significantly ($p < 0.0001$) more often in size (≥1 mm) than had the largest aneurysms in those without any rupture (26 of 26, or 100%, vs 13 of 61, 21%). Those aneurysms that ruptured had also grown significantly ($p < 0.0001$) more than had the largest aneurysms in those without any rupture (6.3 ± 4.2 vs 0.8 ± 1.9 mm; 0.95 ± 1.37 vs 0.04 ± 0.09 mm/yr; or 38.3 ± 72.0 vs 0.9 ± 2.3%/yr) [4].

Current cigarette smoking at end of follow-up and female gender were the only significant independent risk factors for aneurysm growth of ≥1 mm but only current smoking was a risk factor for growth of ≥3 mm [4]. Age adjusted odds ratios are shown in Table 3.

During 1789 patient years of follow-up in 89 patients with unruptured aneurysms, 15 developed a total of 19 de novo aneurysms (2 caused SAH) in locations at which the initial angiography showed no aneurysm. Probability of de novo aneurysm formation cases was 0.84% per year (95% CI, 0.47 to 1.37%) [4]. In addition, there were 5 patients who had no unruptured aneurysms at the beginning of follow-up. They later developed new aneurysms which caused SAH, but these patients survived to undergo angiography. Female gender and current smoking at end of follow-up were the only significant ($p < 0.05$) independent risk factors for de novo aneurysm formation [4]. A logistic

Table 4. *Age- and Hypertension-Adjusted Multivariate Odds Ratios of de Novo Aneurysm Formation*

Characteristic	Odds ratio	95% confidence interval
Female gender	4.73	1.16–19.38*
Current cigarette smoking	4.07	1.09–15.15*

* p < 0.05.

regression model after adjustment for age at diagnosis and definite hypertension is shown in Table 4.

Discussion

Annual rupture rate of 1.3% (95% confidence interval (CI), 0.9% to 1.7%) was similar to all other previously published patient series (1% to 3%) [2, 3, 7–9] but was significantly (p < 0.0001) higher than in the ISUIA (0.3%; 95% CI 0.2% to 0.4%) [6] suggesting that there may be a serious systematic study bias due to failures of inclusion criteria or follow-up of patients in the ISUIA.

A higher incidence of SAH in Finland (13 to 16 per 100.000/yr) [1, 5] as compared to other western countries (ca 10 per 100.000/yr) cannot explain the differences in rupture rates between our study and that of the ISUIA. Among general population aged > 30 years, incidence of SAH is ca 40 to 50 (range 30 to 60) per 100,000 per year [1, 5]. Prevalence of intracranial aneurysms in autopsy and angiographic series among adults ranges between 2% and 5% [2]. Accordingly, risk of rupture of an unruptured aneurysm is between 0.6% and 3% (mean 1.3%) per year. This supports the results of the studies [2, 3, 7–9] on rupture risk of unruptured aneurysms except for the ISUIA [6]. This also suggests that patients with a prior SAH do not have an increased risk for rupture of an unruptured aneurysm although they may have an increased risk for aneurysm formation.

Based on these data, size of aneurysm, age inversely, and current cigarette smoking were independent predictors for subsequent aneurysm rupture. The relative risk of cigarette smoking, tested as a time-dependent covariate, increased if the patient continued smoking during the follow-up. These three risk factors were significant also after adjustment for sex, hypertension, and aneurysm group.

In addition, current cigarette smoking and female gender seem to be factors affecting both aneurysm formation and its growth. Women in particular were at high risk for aneurysm formation, and cigarette smok-

ing hastened growth of pre-existing aneurysm. The faster the growth, the more likely the rupture. Aneurysm size may also be associated with mortality after rupture.

Cigarette smoking has been shown in several studies [3, 4] to increase risk for SAH in all age-groups but the mechanism by which smoking increases this risk has remained unknown. The prevalence of smoking in SAH patients ranges from 45 to 75% whereas in the general adult population it is 20 to 35%. According to findings of this study, it is likely that smoking causes increased risk for SAH by formation of an aneurysm and especially by hastening its growth. Among smoking habits, the number of cigarettes smoked daily seems to be more important concerning aneurysm growth than duration of or age at starting of smoking. In addition, those who had quitted smoking had no increased risk for aneurysm growth. So, cessation of cigarette smoking seems always to be justified for patients with either unruptured aneurysms or prior SAH.

Other recent studies suggest that cigarette smokers' plasma and artery wall elastase/alpha-1-antitrypsin imbalance (i.e. increased elastase activity and/or decreased alpha-1-antitrypsin activity) may contribute either to aneurysm formation or to SAH [3, 4].

Conclusions

Cigarette smoking and female gender seem to be important factors affecting both aneurysm formation and its growth. Age, family history, alcohol consumption, and hypertension each has a lesser impact on this development. In a larger patient population, these factors might also have reached statistical significance. Cessation of smoking is very important for patients with unruptured aneurysms and possibly also for those with a prior SAH. Cessation may also be an alternative to surgery for an unruptured aneurysm, especially in older patients with small aneurysms. However, the author recommend, that unruptured aneurysms should be operated on irrespective of their size and of patients' smoking status, especially in young and middle-aged adults (age < 60 years), if this is technically possible and the patient's concurrent diseases are not contraindications for surgery.

Acknowledgment

This research was supported in part by grants from the Maire Taponen Foundation and the Paavo Nurmi Foundation.

References

1. Fogelholm R, Hernesniemi J, Vapalahti M (1993) Impact of early surgery on outcome after aneurysmal subarachnoid hemorrhage: a population-based study. Stroke 24: 1649–1654
2. Juvela S, Porras M, Heiskanen O (1993). Natural history of unruptured intracranial aneurysms: a long-term follow-up study. J Neurosurg 79: 174–182
3. Juvela S, Porras M, Poussa K (2000) Natural history of unruptured intracranial aneurysms: probability of and risk factors for aneurysm rupture. J Neurosurg 93: 379–387
4. Juvela S, Poussa K, Porras M (2001) Factors affecting formation and growth of intracranial aneurysms: a long-term follow-up study. Stroke 32: 485–491
5. Numminen H, Kotila M, Waltimo O, Aho K, Kaste M (1996) Declining incidence and mortality rates of stroke in Finland from 1972 to 1991. Results of three population-based stroke registers. Stroke 27: 1487–1491
6. The International Study of Unruptured Intracranial Aneurysms Investigators (1998) Unruptured intracranial aneurysms – risk of rupture and risks of surgical intervention. N Engl J Med 339: 1725–1733
7. Wiebers DO, Whisnant JP, Sundt TM Jr, O'Fallon WM (1987) The significance of unruptured intracranial saccular aneurysms. J Neurosurg 66: 23–29
8. Winn HR, Almaani WS, Berga SL, Jane JA, Richardson AE (1983) The long-term outcome in patients with multiple aneurysms: Incidence of late hemorrhage and implications for treatment of incidental aneurysms. J Neurosurg 59: 642–651
9. Yasui N, Suzuki A, Nishimura H, Suzuki K, Abe T (1997) Long-term follow-up study of unruptured intracranial aneurysms. Neurosurgery 40: 1155–1160

Correspondence: Seppo Juvela, M.D., Department of Neurosurgery, Helsinki University Central Hospital, Topeliuksenkatu 5, FIN-00260 Helsinki 26, Finland.

Acta Neurochir (2002) [Suppl] 82: 31–34
© Springer-Verlag 2002

Is the Rupture of Cerebral Berry Aneurysms Influenced by the Perianeurysmal Environment?*

D. San Millán Ruíz[1], K. Tokunaga[1], A. R. Dehdashti[2], K. Sugiu[1], J. Delavelle[1], and D. A. Rüfenacht[1]

[1] Department of Neuroradiology, University of Geneva, Geneva, Switzerland
[2] Department of Neurosurgery – HUG, University of Geneva, Geneva, Switzerland

Summary

Purpose. To evaluate contact between cerebral berry aneurysms and the perianeurysmal environment and to study the influence this contact has on aneurysm rupture.

Materials and Methods. In a series of 76 consecutive patients, pre- and post-contrast CT images of 87 aneurysms were evaluated. Aneurysm locations were identified and aneurysms were divided into two different groups depending on whether they had ruptured or not. Contact between aneurysms and the perianeurysmal environment was studied when present, and considered to be balanced or unbalanced according to symmetry of contact and type of contact interface, i.e. with bone, dura, etc.

Results. Rupture occurred in 47 aneurysms at an average maximum dome size of 7.4 mm. There was contact with elements of the perianeurysmal environment in 38 (81%) of ruptured cases and no evidence of contact in 7 (15%). The nature of contact was unclear in 2 (4%) ruptured aneurysms. In the aneurysms with contact, the nature of contact was unbalanced in 34 (72%) and balanced in 4 (9%). Unbalanced aneurysms ruptured at significantly smaller sizes (average: 7.7 mm) than balanced aneurysms (average: 11.4 mm). Seven aneurysms of small size (3.3–6.9 mm, average: 4.8 mm) were found to have ruptured, despite the fact that they were too small to exhibit contact with the perianeurysmal environment. In 40 unruptured aneurysms (average size: 6.3 mm), contact with the perianeurysmal environment was found in 15 aneurysms, for which balanced contact was found in 11 (27.5%) and unbalanced contact in 4 (10%), and no contact in 25 (62.5%). The average size of the aneurysms without contact (3.7 mm) was significantly smaller than that with balanced contact (10.3 mm) or with unbalanced contact (11.3 mm).

Conclusion. Aneurysms exhibit contact with their perianeurysmal environment as soon as they reach a size that exceeds their allowance given by the local subarachnoid space. The contact with the environment was found to be an additional determinant parameter in the evolution of cerebral berry aneurysms and their risk to rupture.

Keywords: Cerebral aneurysm; unruptured; ruptured; anatomy.

Introduction

Cerebral berry aneurysms are thought to grow typically in circumscribed areas of a weakened arterial wall at the point of arterial bifurcation [12]. Subsequent aneurysm growth is considered to be influenced mainly by blood flow dynamics [2–5, 10–12]. Conditions of aneurysm rupture have been thought to be dominated by morphological criteria including aneurysm size [1, 7, 8, 13, 14], irregularity [3, 12] and wall thickness [11], and by flow and pressure conditions [4, 10].

Cerebral aneurysms develop initially within the free subarachnoid space. As they grow beyond a certain size, they may come into contact with brain, bone, dura, vessels, and cranial nerves, all of which constitute the perianeurysmal environment. These contacts may act as an external influence which may potentially affect aneurysm growth and rupture. The purpose of this study is to evaluate the influence of the perianeurysmal environment on aneurysm rupture.

Materials and Methods

A series of 87 consecutive cerebral berry aneurysms was retrospectively evaluated in 76 patients referred to our hospital over a period of 15 months. In all cases, aneurysm evaluation was based on CT imaging before and after use of an intravenous bolus injection of contrast material (CTA). MR imaging became available for some unruptured cases (15 aneurysms, 37.5%). Additional information was obtained from image reconstruction including 3D representation or reformation in planes allowing for a better evaluation of contact with elements of the perianeurysmal environment.

Aneurysms were classified as ruptured or unruptured depending on the presence or absence of subarachnoid hemorrhage, determined

* Financial support was granted by William COOK Europe A/S, Bjaeverskov, Denmark.

by CT. Aneurysm size was determined for each aneurysm and was defined as the largest diameter at the dome (maximum dome size). Aneurysms were further subdivided by evaluating the interaction between an aneurysm and the perianeurysmal environment. This was achieved by studying the contact between the aneurysm wall and surrounding anatomical elements such as brain, dura, bone, vessels and cranial nerves. Furthermore, contact was arbitrarily qualified as balanced or unbalanced depending on the symmetry of the constraint to which the aneurysm surface was exposed whenever contact was identified. The following conditions were considered to produce an unbalanced contact: 1) the area of contact on the surface of the aneurysm was found to be outside a symmetry line, i.e. contact point on the lateral surface of the aneurysm, and 2) anatomical elements of different nature involved in the contact, i.e. dura on one side and brain on another. If a clear definition of the contact was not possible based on the available imaging studies, type of contact was labeled as unclear.

Unpaired t-test was used for statistical evaluation to compare the average maximum dome sizes among the subgroups.

Results

This study included 87 aneurysms of 76 patients (42 females, 34 males, average age: 53 y/o), in which 47 were ruptured aneurysms and 40 were unruptured. Conditions leading to the diagnosis of 40 unruptured aneurysms included prior episodes of SAH from a concomitant aneurysm in 18 aneurysms, incidental finding in 20 aneurysms, and presence of mass effect in 2 aneurysms. The average dome size measurements for ruptured and unruptured aneurysms were 7.4 mm (range: 2.3–22.9 mm) and 6.3 mm (range: 1.0–30.0 mm), respectively. The size difference between the two groups was not statistically significant.

The distribution of the locations of 47 ruptured aneurysms and their frequency are as follows: 15 middle cerebral artery (MCA) aneurysms, 12 anterior communicating artery (Acom) aneurysms, 8 posterior communicating artery (Pcom) aneurysms, 4 internal carotid (IC) bifurcation aneurysms, 2 anterior choroidal artery (ACho) aneurysms, 2 posterior inferior cerebellar artery (PICA) aneurysms, 1 basilar (BA) tip aneurysm, 1 posterior cerebral artery aneurysm, 1 distal anterior cerebral artery (ACA) aneurysm, and 1 basilar artery-superior cerebellar artery (BA-SCA) aneurysm.

Evaluation of the interactions between ruptured aneurysms and the perianeurysmal environment revealed absence of contact in 7 aneurysms (15%), balanced contact in 4 aneurysms (9%) (Fig. 1), and unbalanced contact in 34 aneurysms (72%). Ruptured aneurysms with no contact were significantly smaller than ruptured aneurysms with contact, with an average maximum dome size of: 4.8 mm versus 8.1 mm

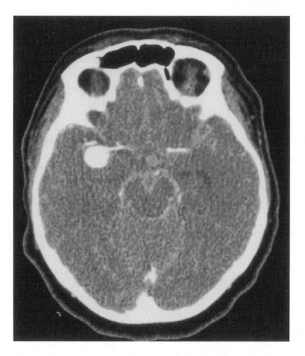

Fig. 1. A source image of three dimensional CT angiography demonstrating a middle cerebral aneurysm with a maximum dome size of 15.0 mm with "balanced" contact with the perianeurysmal environment

(P < 0.02). Among the ruptured aneurysms with contact, the average maximum dome size for those with unbalanced contact was significantly smaller than those with balanced contact (7.8 mm versus 11.4 mm; P < 0.05). The nature of contact was unclear in 2 (4%) ruptured aneurysms.

The distribution and frequency of the locations of the 40 unruptured aneurysms are summarized as follows: 17 aneurysms at MCA, 5 at IC ophthalmic artery, 5 at ACho, 3 at a superior hypophyseal artery, 3 at Acom, 2 at Pcom, 2 at BA tip, 1 at distal ACA, 1 at IC bifurcation, and 1 BA-SCA.

Evaluation of the interactions between unruptured aneurysms and the perianeurysmal environment revealed presence of contact in 15 aneurysms (37.5%), absence of contact in 25 aneurysms (62.5%). Contact was found to be balanced in 11 aneurysms (27.5%) and unbalanced in 4 aneurysms (10%) (Fig. 2). Unruptured aneurysms without contact had a significantly smaller average maximum dome size (average: 3.6 mm) than those with balanced contact (average: 10.3 mm) (P < 0.005) or with unbalanced contact (average: 11.3 mm) (P < 0.005). There were no significant differences in terms of size between the group with balanced contact and that with unbalanced contact.

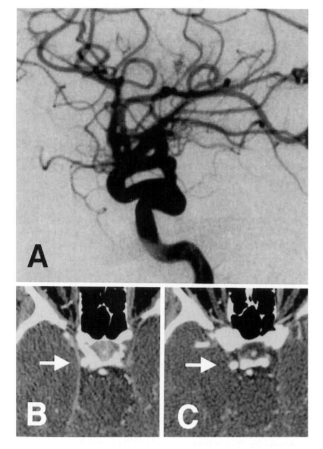

Fig. 2. (A) A right internal carotid angiogram showing a postero-inferiorly oriented posterior communicating artery aneurysm with a maximum dome size of 9.5 mm. (B, C) Source images of three dimensional CT angiography demonstrating the aneurysm (arrow) with "unbalanced" contact with the bone, the tentorial edge, and the temporal lobe

Discussion

Although aneurysm size has been reported to be the significant predicting factor for the risk of aneurysm rupture [7], several publications have revealed the difficulty of accepting that aneurysm size alone should be applied when assessing the risk of aneurysm rupture [1, 2, 6, 8, 9, 11, 12]. Several factors are currently considered as influencing the growth and rupture of aneurysms. Such parameters include blood flow hemodynamics that act from within the aneurysm [4, 10], or wall strength which may play a key role in the risk of aneurysm rupture, but which remains difficult to assess in vivo [11]. However, the role of external parameters influencing the aneurysm growth and rupture has been largely ignored. Cerebral aneurysms grow within the subarachnoid space, a space that is traversed by cranial nerves, vessels, and arachnoid trabe-

culae, and is bounded by brain, dura, and bone. These anatomical elements form the perianeurysmal environment, and may come to interact with the aneurysm wall as soon as the aneurysm grows beyond a certain size. This study attempted in evaluating the interaction between an aneurysm and the perianeurysmal environment by identifying the existance of contact between the aneurysm wall and the surrounding elements. The purpose was to then assess whether interactions between the perianeurysmal environment and an aneurysm may influence the rate of aneurysm rupture.

Interestingly enough, there was no significant difference in average maximum dome sizes between ruptured and unruptured aneurysms (7.4 mm versus 6.3 mm). Contact with anatomical elements of the environment was present both in ruptured and unruptured aneurysms. However, ruptured aneurysms exhibited contact with the environment more frequently than unruptured aneurysms (81% versus 37.5%). Furthermore, the rate of unbalanced contact was superior for ruptured aneurysms than for unruptured aneurysms (72% versus 10%). Unbalanced contact was the most frequent form of contact between ruptured aneurysms and their environment, whilst balanced contact was the most frequent in unruptured aneurysms.

These results suggest that presence of contact between an aneurysm and elements of the perianeurysmal environment is associated with higher rates and, therefore, higher risk of aneurysm rupture, and that this risk is further elevated if contact occurs in an unbalanced fashion. Aneurysm size probably influences risk of aneurysm rupture in as much as large size increases the probability for an aneurysm to establish contact with an anatomical element of the perianeurysmal environment. As the perianeurysmal environment changes morphologically according to the subarachnoid cistern in which the aneurysm develops, location of the aneurysm will also need to be assessed for determining risk of rupture in terms of aneurysm size. This aspect deserves to be further explored.

A special subgroup of aneurysm appears in the form of ruptured aneurysm that didn't exhibit contact (15%) (Fig. 3). These aneurysms were significantly smaller than ruptured aneurysms that exhibited contact (4.8 mm versus 8.1 mm maximum dome size, $P < 0.02$). Weak wall structure could explain why these aneurysms rupture at smaller sizes before they become submitted to the external influences of the perianeurysmal environment.

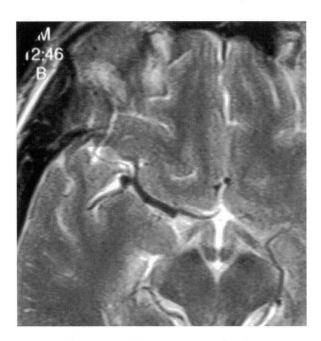

Fig. 3. A T2 weighted MR image on an axial view showing a right middle cerebral artery aneurysm with a maximum dome size of 3.0 mm without any contact with the adjacent anatomical structures

Conclusion

It is difficult to assess the risk of aneurysm rupture based on size only. The perianeurysmal environment was found to have a significant impact on aneurysmal rupture. Aneurysms exhibit contact with their perianeurysmal environment as soon as they reach a size that exceeds their allowance given by the local subarachnoid space. The contact with the environment was found to be an additional determinant parameter in the evolution of cerebral berry aneurysms and their risk to rupture. Ruptured aneurysms too small to develop contact with elements of the perianeurysmal environment, probably rupture because of weak aneurysm wall.

References

1. Asari S, Ohmoto T (1993) Natural history and risk factors of unruptured cerebral aneurysms. Clin Neurol Neurosurg 95: 205–214
2. Crompton MR (1966) Mechanism of growth and rupture in cerebral berry aneurysms. Br Med J 1: 1138–1142
3. Ferguson GG (1972) Physical factors in the initiation, growth, and rupture of human intracranial saccular aneurysms. J Neurosurg 37: 666–677
4. Gonzalez CF, Cho YI, Ortega HV, Moret J (1992) Intracranial aneurysms: flow analysis of their origin and progression. AJNR Am J Neuroradiol 13: 181–188
5. Hashimoto N, Handa H, Nagata I, Hazama F (1983) Saccular cerebral aneurysms in rats. Am J Pathol 110: 397–399
6. Inagawa T, Hirano A (1990) Ruptured intracranial aneurysms: an autopsy study of 133 patients. Surg Neurol 33: 117–123
7. International Study of Unruptured Intracranial Aneurysms Investigators (1998) Unruptured intracranial aneurysms – risk of rupture and risks of surgical intervention. N Engl J Med 339: 1725–1733
8. Juvela S, Porras M, Heiskanen O (1993) Natural history of unruptured intracranial aneurysms: a long-term follow-up study. J Neurosurg 79: 174–182
9. Rinkel GJ, Djibuti M, van Gijn J (1998) Prevalence and risk of rupture of intracranial aneurysms: a systematic review. Stroke 29: 251–256
10. Stehbens WE (1989) Etiology of intracranial berry aneurysms. J Neurosurg 70: 823–831
11. Suzuki J, Ohara H (1978) Clinicopathological study of cerebral aneurysms. Origin, rupture, repair, and growth. J Neurosurg 48: 505–514
12. Weir B (1987) Aneurysms affecting the nervous system. Chapter 5 pathology. Williams & Wilkins Baltimore, pp 209–261
13. Wiebers DO, Whisnant JP, O'Fallon WM (1981) The natural history of unruptured intracranial aneurysms. N Engl J Med 304: 696–698
14. Wiebers DO, Whisnant JP, Sundt TM, Jr, O'Fallon WM (1987) The significance of unruptured intracranial saccular aneurysms. J Neurosurg 66: 23–29

Correspondence: Daniel A. Rüfenacht, Neuroradiology – HUG, University of Geneva, 24 rue Micheli-du-Crest, 1211 Geneva 14, Switzerland.

Acta Neurochir (2002) [Suppl] 82: 35–39

Surgical Prognosis of Unruptured Cerebral Aneurysms. Report of 40 Cases in University Hospital Zurich

H. Ishihara, S. Yoshimura, L. Könü, N. Khan, and **Y. Yonekawa**

Department of Neurosurgery, University Hospital Zurich, Zurich, Switzerland

Summary

A series of 40 patients admitted to University Hospital Zurich (1996~97) with unruptured cerebral aneurysms is reported. Fifty-two aneurysms were treated in 40 operations. The age of surgically treated patients ranged from 31 to 78 year old (mean 53.6). The main locations of the aneurysms were: MCA 21 (40.4%), AcomA 10 (19.2%), ICA (posterior communicating and bifurcation) 6 (11.5%), carotid-ophthalmic segment 4 (7.7%), ACA 4 (7.7%), basilar tip 3 (5.8%), vertebral artery 2 (3.8%). The circumstances of diagnosis were: incidental 15 (37.5%), other cranial lesions 9 (22.5%), symptomatic 8 (20%), multiple aneurysm 8 (20%). The overall outcome of surgery was: good recovery in 39 cases (97.5%), moderately disabled in 1 case (2.5%) who was 56 year-old and had three aneurysms including basilar tip. There was no operative mortality. Though this series has small number of patients, it suggests that location of the aneurysm is an important factor affecting surgical outcome among patient age, the circumstances of the diagnosis, size and location of aneurysm.

Keywords: Cerebral aneurysm; unruptured aneurysm; surgical treatment; basilar head aneurysm.

Abbreviations

ACA Anterior cerebral artery
AcomA anterior communicating artery
ICA internal carotid artery
MCA middle cerebral artery
PcomA posterior communicating artery

Introduction

Together with progression in neuroimaging techniques like magnetic resonance imaging (MRI), magnetic resonance angiography (MRA), and computed tomographic angiography (CTA), unruptured cerebral aneurysms have been revealed with increasing frequency. Because of the high mortality and morbidity rate in patients with subarachnoid hemorrhage, most of the unruptured aneurysms have been operated. However, the International Study of Unruptured Intracranial Aneurysms has cast questions on the surgical treatment of unruptured aneurysms [1], although several criticisms exist. Since surgical treatment for unruptured intracranial aneurysms is warranted if the risk of its natural history is greater than the risk of surgery, it is required to accumulate data of its natural history as well as surgical results. Also, the further improvement of surgical techniques are required.

We report the surgical outcome of 40 patients with unruptured intracranial aneurysms in University Hospital Zurich. The strategies for basilar bifurcation aneurysm were discussed.

Patients and Methods

Between 1996 and 1997, 247 patients with intracranial aneurysms underwent microsurgical treatment in the Department of Neurosurgery at University Hospital Zurich. Of these, 40 patients were unruptured aneurysm cases. There were 21 (52.5%) women with an average age of 56.4 years and 19 (47.5%) men with an average of 50.5 years.

The surgical outcomes were assessed 3 to 6 months after operation. The patients were graded with Glasgow Outcome Score (GOS).

Results

The age of patients ranged from 31 to 78 years. The distribution of age was, less than 40 years (5 patients), 40 to 49 years (9 patients), 50 to 59 years (13 patients), 60 to 69 years (11 patients), and more than 70 years (2 patients).

The circumstances of diagnosis are described in Table 1. In this series, when the relation between the symptom and aneurysm was not clear, the aneurysm was regarded as incidental. Most of the incidental aneurysms were diagnosed after examination for headache or dizziness.

Table 1. *Circumstances of Diagnosis*

1. Multiple aneurysms*	8 (20%)
2. Unrelated intracranial lesion	9 (22.5%)
brain tumor [2]	
intracranial hemorrhage [1]	
ischemic cerebrovascular disease [6]	
3. Symptomatic aneurysm	8 (20%)
mass effect [1]	
ischemic stroke [3]	
headache [3]	
4. Incidental aneurysm	15 (37.5%)

* Multiple aneurysms mean unruptured aneurysms discovered after subarachnoid hemorrhage.

Table 2. *Location and Size of Aneurysms in 40 Patients with 52 Unruptured Aneurysms*

		2–5 mm	6–9 mm	10–14 mm	15–24 mm	25 mm
MCA	21 (40.4%)	10	8	1	2	
ACA	14 (26.9%)	8	5	1		
ICA	12 (23.1%)	3	7		1	1
BA-tip	3 (5.8%)		2	1		
VA	2 (3.8%)		1	1		
Total	52 (100%)	21	23	4	3	1

Fifty-two aneurysms were microsurgically treated in 40 patients. The size and location of aneurysms are summarised in Table 2. The locations of aneurysms were at: the MCA 21 (40.4%), the ACA 14 (26.9%) (AcomA 10, distal ACA 8), the ICA 12 (23.1%) (PcomA and bifurcation 6, carotid-ophthalmic segment 4, cavernous segment 2), basilar tip 3 (5.8%), the vertebral artery 2 (3.8%). The aneurysms which were less than 10 mm in diameter accounted for 44 (84.6 %). There were 4 aneurysms which were more than 15 mm in diameter. Two of them were located on cavernous portion of the ICA, and they were treated by trapping and EC-IC bypass. The other two were located on MCA.

The surgical outcomes assessed at 3 to 6 months later were; Good recovery in 39 patients (97.5%), Moderately disabled in 1 patient (2.5%). There was no severely disabled case, nor was there any surgical mortality.

Presentation of a Single Case with Morbidity

A 57 year-old man developed transient numbness in his left arm. Although the cause of the symptom was not detected, aneurysms were found on CT. He was admitted to our department on January 13, 1997. A neurological examination at admission revealed no neurological symptoms. Angiographies showed three aneurysms located at the AcomA, right MCA and basilar tip. The size of basilar bifurcation aneurysm was 7 mm in diameter, and the neck was located 4 mm above the posterior clinoid process (Fig. 1). A conventional right pterional craniotomy was followed by extra dural selective anterior clinoidectomy. Anterior communicating artery aneurysm was clipped at first.

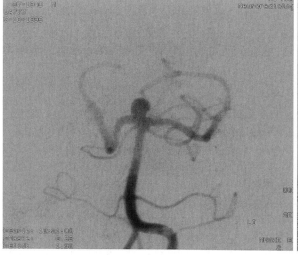
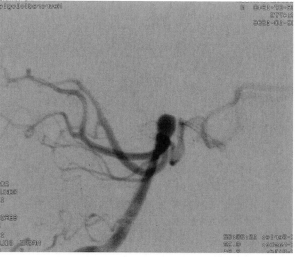

a   **b**

Fig. 1. Case 57-year-old man. (a) AP view. (b) Lateral view

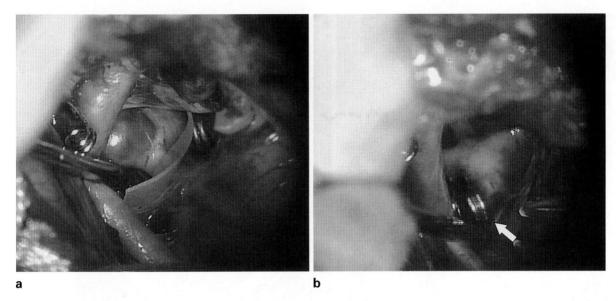

Fig. 2. Operative findings. (a) Before permanent clipping. Note temporary clipping on basilar trunk, and isolation of aneurysm from perforators with a rubber dam. (b) After permanent clipping. Note translocation of the PcomA

Then, basilar tip aneurysm was treated through retro-carotid space. After temporary clipping of basilar trunk, the aneurysm was isolated from thalamoperforating arteries with a rubber dam, and clipped. After confirming complete clipping, the dome was punctured and the preservation of thalamoperforators was confirmed from both sides of P1 segment. Also, the preservation of the PcomA and anterior choroidal artery was confirmed, but the PcomA was slightly translocated upwards (Fig. 2). Finally, the MCA aneurysm was also clipped. Postoperatively, this patient developed moderate left hemiparesis which was predominant in upper limb. A CT scan revealed a small infarction in posterior limb of right internal capsule (Fig. 3). After 3 months of the neuro-rehabilitation, he is leading his life independently.

Discussion

Among 40 patients who were microsurgically treated with unruptured intracranial aneurysms, surgical morbidity was observed in one patient with a basilar tip aneurysm. This result suggests that the location of aneurysm, especially basilar tip aneurysm, is an important factor influencing surgical outcome.

Although there are some controversies, several reports have shown higher surgical morbidity and mortality in posterior circulation aneurysms. Orz *et al.* investigated 310 patients with incidental intracranial aneurysms, and they observed a 28% morbidity and mortality with surgical treatment of posterior circulation aneurysms compared to a 12% for anterior circulation aneurysms [3]. Khanna *et al.* analyzed 172 unruptured aneurysm cases, and they also found that the location of aneurysm in posterior circulation was associated with higher incidence of poor outcome independent of the aneurysm size. They established an unruptured aneurysm risk classification including the location of aneurysm [2]. On the other hand, Solomon *et al.* reported that only the size of aneurysm was associated with surgical risk except for giant basilar aneurysms [7]. However, even in the latter study, the surgical morbidity was high in giant basilar aneurysm, suggesting that the location of aneurysm was associated with surgical outcome.

In order to prevent surgical morbidity, surgical strategies are necessary for treating individual aneurysms. The fundamental surgical strategy for unruptured basilar tip aneurysms and basilar artery-superior cerebellar artery aneurysms in our institute is as follows:

1. Conventional pterional craniotomy, usually from the right side.
2. Selective extradural anterior clinoidectomy [11]

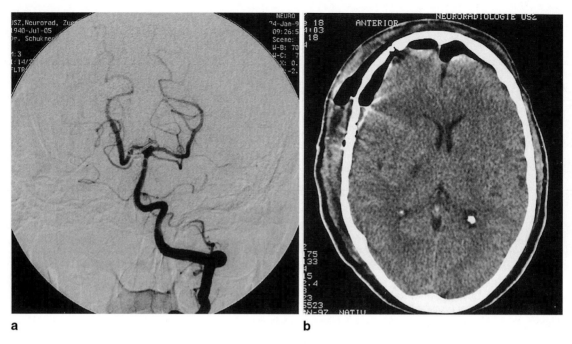

Fig. 3. (a) Postoperative angiography, AP view, showing occlusion of the aneurysm and preservation of thalamoperforating arteries from P1 segments. (b) Postoperative CT scan shows an infarction in right posterior limb of internal capsule

3. Minimum opening of cisterns. (the prevention of postoperative hygroma)
4. Posterior clinoidectomy, when it's required
5. Temporary clipping of the BA trunk
6. Isolation of the aneurysm from perforators with a rubber dam
7. Permanent clipping of the aneurysm and puncture of its dome.

Needless to say, this strategy is premised on individual preoperative evaluations including the characters of aneurysm and its relation with surrounding structures [10].

Selective extradural anterior clinoidectomy is an additional technique to pterional approach, and it is considered a useful procedure for treatment of basilar tip aneurysm. In this technique, anterior clinoid process is removed, the lateral and superior wall of the entire optic canal is unroofed, and optic sheath and distal dural ring are opened [11]. The ICA and optic nerve are mobilized by using this technique, and as a result, retrocarotid space and also opticocarotid triangle are widened. This technique is also greatly useful for treatment of paraclinoid aneurysms.

In this series, a postoperative neurological deficit was seen in a patient with basilar tip aneurysm. The lesion was an infarction in posterior limb of internal capsule. The territories of the basal perforating arteries varies with the individual. The anterior segment of the posterior limb of the internal capsule can be supplied by the thalamotuberal artery or anterior choroidal artery at the axial level of midthalamus [5, 9]. Operative findings and postoperative angiography didn't indicate the occlusion of the anterior choroidal artery, the PcomA nor the thalamoperforators from the posterior cerebral artery. Since the PcomA was retracted to treat basilar tip aneurysm and slightly translocated after permanent clipping, a possible explanation for this infarction was distortion of the thalamotuberal artery. Since the existence and diameter of the perforating arteries are relatively constant regardless of the diameter of the PcomA [3, 8], the thalamotuberal artery must be given attention during the approach to basilar tip aneurysm even if the PcomA is hypoplastic [6].

A large number of critical perforating arteries are involved in surgical treatment especially for basilar tip aneurysm, and their retraction for surgical manipulation and their slight translocation by aneurysm clipping itself can cause impairment of microcirculations even though they are not directly damaged. This may account for the higher surgical morbidity rate in basilar tip aneurysm.

Conclusion

The surgical morbidity of unruptured aneurysm was 2.5% in our institute. Location of aneurysm was associated with surgical risk in this series. It is considered that higher surgical risk in basilar tip aneurysm is due to vital basal perforating arteries.

Acknowledgment

The authors thank Mr. Peter Roth, Mr. Andre Roth and Ms. Rosmarie Frick for their assistance.

References

1. International Study of Unruptured Intracranial Aneurysms Investigators (1998) Unruptured intracranial aneurysms. Risk of rupture and risks of surgical intervention. N Engl J Med 339: 1725–1733
2. Khanna RK, Malik GM, Qureshi N (1996) Predicting outcome following surgical treatment of unruptured intracranial aneurysms: a proposed grading system. J Neurosurg 84: 49–54
3. Orz YI, Hongo K, Tanaka Y, Nagashima H, Osawa M, Kyoshima K, Kobayashi S (2000) Risks of surgery for patients with unruptured intracranial aneurysms. Surg Neurol 53: 21–29
4. Pedroza A, Dujovny M, Artero JC, Umansky F, Berman K, Diaz FG, Ausman JI, Mirchandani HG (1987) Microanatomy of the posterior communicating artery. Neurosurgery 20: 228–235
5. Pullicino PM (1993) The course and territories of cerebral small arteries. Adv Neurol 62: 11–39
6. Regli L, de Tribolet N (1991) Tuberothalamic infarct after division of a hypoplastic posterior communicating artery for clipping of a basilar tip aneurysm. Case report. Neurosurgery 28: 456–459
7. Solomon RA, Fink ME, Pile-Spellman J (1994) Surgical management of unruptured intracranial aneurysms. J Neurosurg 80: 440–446
8. Takahashi S, Goto K, Fukasawa H, Kawata Y, Uemura K, Yaguchi K (1985) Computed tomography of cerebral infarction along the distribution of the basal perforating arteries. Part II: thalamic arterial group. Radiology 155: 119–130
9. Vincentelli F, Caruso G, Grisoli F, Rabehanta P, Andriamamonjy C, Gouaze A (1990) Microsurgical anatomy of the cisternal course of the perforating branches of the posterior communicating artery. Neurosurgery 26: 824–831
10. Yonekawa Y, Kaku Y, Imhof H-G, Kiss M, Curcic M, Taub E, Roth P (1999) Posterior circulation aneurysms. Technical strategies based on angiographic anatomical findings and the results of 60 recent consecutive cases. Acta Neurochir (Wien) [Suppl] 72: 123–140
11. Yonekawa Y, Ogata N, Imhof H-G, Olivecrona M, Strommer K, Kwak TE, Roth P, Groscurth P (1997) Selective extradural anterior clinoidectomy for supra- and parasellar processes. Technical note. J Neurosurg 87: 636–642

Correspondence: H. Ishihara, Department of Neurosurgery, University Hospital Zurich, Frauenklinikstr. 10, CH-8091 Zurich, Switzerland.

Acta Neurochir (2002) [Suppl] 82: 41–46
© Springer-Verlag 2002

Endovascular Coiling Compared with Surgical Clipping for the Treatment of Unruptured Middle Cerebral Artery Aneurysms: An Update

L. Regli[1], **A. R. Dehdashti**[2], **A. Uske**[1], and **N. de Tribolet**[2]

[1] Department of Neurosurgery and Radiology, Centre Hospitalier Universitaire Vaudois, Lausanne, Switzerland
[2] Department of Neurosurgery, Hôpitaux Universitaires Genève, Geneva, Switzerland

Summary

Object. In 1999 we reported that 94% of unruptured middle cerebral artery (MCA) aneurysms managed prospectively between 1993 and 1997, according to a protocol favoring endovascular coiling, were best treated by surgical clipping. The goal of the current study was to delineate the most appropriate treatment option for unruptured MCA aneurysms today, considering the technical advances in imaging and in endovascular treatment.

Methods. 35 consecutive patients harboring 40 unruptured MCA aneurysms were treated between 1997 and December 2000. Patients with unruptured cerebral aneurysms are managed prospectively according to the same protocol as reported previously [1]: the primary treatment recommendation is endovascular packing with Guglielmi detachable coils (GDCs). Surgical clipping is recommended after failed attempt at coil placement or in the presence of angioanatomical features that contraindicate that type of endovascular therapy.

Results. One unruptured MCA aneurysm was treated by endovascular embolization, 37 unruptured MCA aneurysms were clipped, whereas 2 unruptured MCA aneurysms were trapped with simultaneous extracranial-intracranial revascularization. Postoperative angiography revealed complete exclusion of all aneurysms. Preservation of vascular permeability was demonstrated in all clip-reconstructed aneurysms, despite arterial branches frequently originating from the aneurysmal base. Cerebral revascularization of the distal MCA was successful in the 2 patients with giant aneurysms. None of the patients presented permanent disabling complications from the treatment of the unruptured MCA aneurysm.

Conclusion. Despite major technical advances in imaging and in endovascular treatment of cerebral aneurysms, surgical clipping still is the most efficient treatment for unruptured MCA aneurysms at the beginning of the new millennium.

Keywords: Unruptured cerebral aneurysms; surgical clipping endovascular coiling; middle cerebral artery aneurysm.

Introduction

Management choices in patients with unruptured intracranial aneurysms remain controversial as the natural history of unruptured intracranial aneurysms still is a matter of debate [2, 10, 19, 25]. The decision whether to treat a patient with an unruptured aneurysm depends ultimately on the risk of rupture compared with the risk associated with treatment. A cumulative rate of aneurysm rupture of 1% to 1.3% per year is currently accepted, but rates varying between 0.05% and 2.7% per year have been reported with a case/fatality rate among patients with initially unruptured aneurysms and subsequent hemorrhage as high as 83% [1, 4, 5, 7, 26, 27].

The goal of aneurysm treatment is complete, immediate, permanent, and safe occlusion of the base of the aneurysm with preservation of the parent artery and its branches. Endovascular embolization of cerebral aneurysms is gaining favor as an attractive alternative to surgical clipping [15, 22, 24]. The major factors predicting the success rate of surgical clipping of an unruptured aneurysm are: 1) dome size; 2) aneurysm location; 3) patient age. The major factors predicting the success rate of endovascular coil placement are: 1) endovascular accessibility; 2) ratio between aneurysm dome and neck; 3) aneurysm shape.

Middle cerebral artery aneurysms are frequently associated with multiple intracranial aneurysms, leading to the discovery of a large number of unruptured middle cerebral artery (MCA) aneurysms. They typically have a wide base, and often incorporate the origin of the arterial M2 branches into their base. The authors have reported a consecutive series of unruptured MCA aneurysms treated between 1993 and 1997 and shown that surgical clipping was by far the most efficient treatment option [21]. The purpose of the current study was to update this series and to determine the most

Table 1. *Angioanatomical Features that Contraindicate Endovascular Coil Placement in our Management Protocol*

Neck width > 4 mm
Dome/neck ratio ≤ 1.5
Inadequate endovascular access
Intraluminal thrombus
Arterial branch origin incorporated w/aneurysm neck

appropriate treatment option for unruptured MCA aneurysms today, taking into account the tremendous advances in imaging technology and in endovascular techniques since we reported our previous series.

Materials and Methods

Between July 1997 and December 2000, 35 patients with 40 unruptured MCA aneurysms were evaluated in our department, and constitute the reported series.

Patients who present at our institutions with unruptured MCA aneurysms are managed according to the same protocol as already reported [21]: whenever feasible, our primary recommendation is endovascular treatment by means of GDCs. The presence of an aneurysm is confirmed using CT angiography and intraarterial cerebral angiography. The angioanatomy of the aneurysm is selectively studied using rotational three dimensional (3-D) angiography. These films are then reviewed by the endovascular neuroradiologist along with the vascular neurosurgeons during a weekly cerebrovascular conference. The decision is based on the following criteria: if the vascular anatomy does not contraindicate an endovascular treatment (Table 1), we recommend that supraselective catheterization be performed and GDC coiling be attempted. The complete occlusion of the aneurysm is then confirmed by follow-up control angiogram. Surgical clipping is performed only if patients either are not eligible for aneurysm embolization or if the attempt for coiling fails. Postoperative control angiogram is performed to assure complete occlusion of the aneurysm.

The 40 unruptured MCA aneurysms reported in this series were divided into three groups: Group A consisted of aneurysms successfully treated by embolization; Group B consisted of those aneurysms in which attempts at embolization failed and for which elective surgery was required for clipping; Group C consisted of lesions primarily treated with elective clipping because the angioanatomy of the aneurysm was clearly unsuitable for embolization.

The patient's outcome was recorded according to the Glasgow Outcome Scale [6], which uses the following criteria: 5) excellent (returned to preoperative functional level and employment, with no new neurological deficit); 4) good (minor new neurological deficit that does not interfere with daily activities and employment); 3) fair (significant neurological deficit that interferes with daily activities and prevents return to employment, even if related to preexisting neurological deficit); 2) poor (coma or severe neurological deficit rendering the patient totally dependent); and 1) death.

Results

The characteristics of the 35 patients with 40 unruptured aneurysms of the MCA are detailed in Table 2.

Table 2. *Characteristics of 35 Patients with 40 Unruptured Aneurysms of the MCA*

Characteristics	Value
Patient characteristics	
– Male/female ratio	18/17
– Mean age (years)	50 ± 11
– Mode of presentation	
SAH (from other aneurysm)	17
Incidental*	19
Partial seizures	1
Familial screening**	3
Aneurysm characteristics	
Location	
– MCA bifurcation	33
– M1 segment	6
– M2 segment	1
Size	
– <6 mm	23
– 6–10 mm	13
– 11–25 mm	3
– >25 mm	1
– Mean size (mm)	7.1 ± 6
Multiple intracranial aneurysms	20 (50%)
Bilateral MCA aneurysms (mirror)	6 (15%)

* These patients presented with unrelated signs and symptoms (vertigo, headache). Four patients had ischemic strokes unrelated to the MCA aneurysm (3 from cervical carotid stenosis and 1 from a contralateral carotid bifurcation aneurysm that was coiled).
** One had ploycystic kidney disease.

Group A

One unruptured MCA aneurysm (2%) was treated using GDCs, and was completely excluded from the cerebral circulation in one session. This aneurysm measured 5 mm in diameter and the dome/neck ratio was 3, indicating a narrow neck and predicting a favorable angioanatomy for GDC placement.

Group B

There were no patients in this group in the current series. No unruptured MCA aneurysms underwent an attempt at embolization that failed.

Group C

In 39 unruptured MCA aneurysms (98%) primary surgical treatment was performed, since the neuroradiological evaluation revealed an unfavorable angioanatomy for endovascular treatment. Primary clipping was performed in 37 aneurysms (93%). All had complete aneurysmal occlusion with preservation of

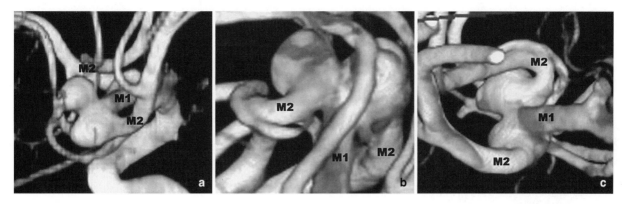

Fig. 1. Rotational 3D intra-arterial angiography showing an unruptured MCA aneurysm from different viewing angles (a, b, c). The images clearly show that the aneurysm has two distinct domes and that the base is very large incorporating the origin of both M2 segments

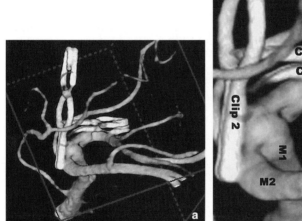
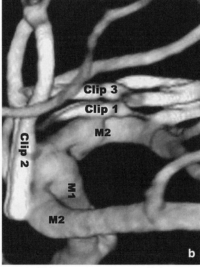

Fig. 2. Post-operative rotational 3D intra-arterial angiography of aneurysm shown in Fig. 1 (a) The complex angioanatomy of the aneurysm necessitated 3 clips for complete exclusion of the aneurysm with reconstruction of both M2 segments (b). Clip 1 is a curved mini-clip, clip 2 is a fenestrated straight clip, and clip 3 is a straight mini-clip the tips of which are in the fenestration of clip 2. Note that both M2 branches have normal permeability. Endovascular reconstruction would not have been possible

the MCA permeability confirmed by post-operative angiography (Figs. 1 and 2).

In two unruptured MCA aneurysms the origin of the M2 arterial segments was incorporated within the aneurysmal wall, therefore trapping with EC-IC bypass was performed. One was a giant saccular aneurysm of 35 mm and the other was a fusiform MCA bifurcation aneurysm of 17 mm. Both aneurysms were completely excluded and the distal MCA was successfully revascularized with superficial temporal artery to M2 middle cerebral artery bypass (Figure 3).

The 3D rotational cerebral angiography was extremely helpful to show accurate angioanatomical features of the aneurysms. In all 39 aneurysms it revealed either a wide base or an arterial branch origin incorporated into the base.

Overall Results

Of 40 unruptured MCA aneurysms, only one (2%) was successfully embolized by GDCs, 37 (93%) were clipped primarily, and 2 (5%) were primarily trapped (the preoperative plan was trapping in combination with revascularization). No patient underwent an embolization attempt that failed. Similarly, no primary surgical treatment plan failed. The fact that all treatment plans succeeded, without failed treatment attempt, is of importance, as this reduces the overall risk of treatment.

Complication and Outcome

There were no complications associated with endovascular treatment. There were two transient compli-

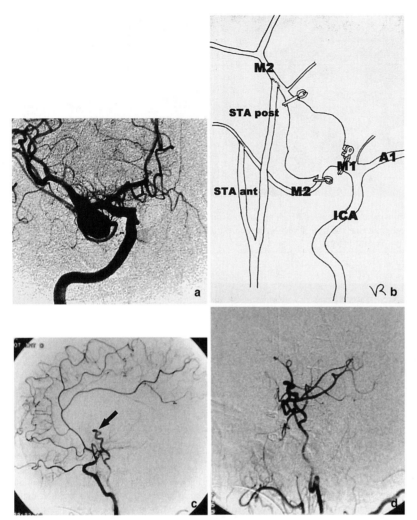

Fig. 3. Large fusiforme MCA aneurysm. Both M2 branches originate from the aneurysmal dome contraindicating clip and coil treatment (a). Patient had double barrel superior temporal artery – middle cerebral artery bypass and trapping (b, schematic representation). Lateral internal carotid artery angiogram demonstrates the filling defect of the MCA branches through the internal carotid artery (c). Some contrast reflux into the external carotid artery shows the superficial temporal artery feeding the bypass (arrow). Selective external carotid artery injection (d) demonstrates the superficial temporal artery filling the MCA territory through the double barrel bypass. Patient had normal postoperative neurological examination

cations (5%) in the surgical group consisting of one patient that developed a chronic subdural hematoma and one patient that presented a psychiatric decompensation with a severe depressive syndrome. The patient with the subdural hematoma recovered normal neurological examination after surgical drainage. The patient with the depressive syndrome had favorable evolution with adequate treatment. Permanent worsening was present in one patient (2.5%) with a giant (35 mm) that had trapping and EC-IC bypass. He presented postoperatively mass effect from the acute thrombosis of the aneurysm and from an intraparenchymal hematoma that needed to be drained. At one year follow-up he had resumed normal daily activities and the same employment despite minor new neurological deficit.

Overall outcome (Table 3) at one year of treatment of 40 unruptured MCA aneurysms was very favorable

Table 3. *Outcome of 35 Patients Treated for 40 Unruptured MCA Aneurysms*

Outcome (Glasgow outcome score)*	Patients
Excellent & good (5–4)	27
Fair (3)	7
Poor (2)	1
Death (1)	0

* Glasgow outcome scores of 3 to 1 were always a consequence of a subarachnoid hemorrhage from another aneurysm.

with no mortality and one (2.5%) permanent neurological worsening, this patient still had a score of 4 on the Glasgow Outcome Scale. Neurological deficits in patients with lower outcome scores were related to sequels to subarachnoid hemorrhage from another ruptured aneurysm and not to treatment of the unruptured MCA aneurysm.

Discussion

Treatment of unruptured intracranial aneurysms should only be recommended if the risk associated with observation outweighs the risk associated with treatment. We recommend the reader to review the data on the natural history of unruptured intracranial aneurysms presented in this Proceedings as this is beyond the scope of our report.

It is our belief that in selected patients treatment of unruptured aneurysms offers considerable benefit if the treatment is safe and efficient. Choosing the treatment modality that provides the best safety and efficacy is an important therapeutic decision, especially for prophylactic therapies. The criteria for choosing between endovascular embolization and microsurgical clipping as a treatment for intracranial aneurysm are not well established. The advantage of studying unruptured aneurysm is that they form a more homogenous group and there is less bias due to different clinical grades. Our protocol for unruptured aneurysm is to recommend endovascular treatment with GDCs whenever feasible and to perform microsurgical clipping only in patients in whom GDC treatment failed or who are excluded from GDC embolization for obvious angioanatomical reasons. Our prior study, including patients treated between 1993 and 1997 [21], was the first publication comparing surgical clipping and endovascular coiling with a protocol favoring coiling and is in contrast with most of the reports that reserved endovascular treatment for poor surgical candidates. We were able to show that 94% (32/34) of unruptured MCA aneurysms had to be treated surgically, 32% failed embolization and 62% had obvious angioanatomical contraindications for embolization. Only 15% (2/11) of the endovascular occlusion attempts succeeded.

The goal of the current study was to verify if these conclusions are still true in light of the technical advances in imaging and in endovascular treatment. The present study shows that in a consecutive series of patients with unruptured MCA aneurysms treated since 1997: 1) only one aneurysm was treated by embolization and 39 (98%) were treated surgically; 2) despite difficult angioanatomical features surgical treatment of MCA aneurysms can be performed with a low rate (2.5%) of permanent morbidity; and 3) better visualization of angioanatomical details with preoperative imaging reduces the rate of treatment failures.

Despite new imaging techniques and refinements

in endovascular coiling, the results of treatment of unruptured MCA aneurysms have not changed compared to our previous results [21]. Unruptured MCA aneurysm are still a major challenge for endovascular surgeons since their base is often wide and incorporates the origin of one or both M2 segments. The remodeling technique applied to the treatment of wide necked aneurysms has allowed to occlude some aneurysms that could not have been treated using the classic GDC technique [12, 13, 16, 17]. However, we share the opinion that remodeling technique should not be attempted in aneurysms of the middle cerebral arteries unless surgical clipping is contraindicated [17].

New refinement in endovascular techniques will continue to improve the results of aneurysm treatment. It is our impression, however, that 3-D rotational angiography reveals the angioanatomy of aneurysms in such detail that it can demonstrate anatomical features unfavorable for coiling that were not seen before on 2D angiography. A wide base incorporating arterial branches can better be seen on 3D images. Surgical clipping is a more versatile technique than coiling and allows reconstruction of a wide aneurysmal base despite the incorporation of arterial branches. Some angioanatomical features contraindicate clipping and necessitate trapping with bypass as done in 2 cases in our series. An important fact is that accurate 3D images can limit unsuccessful attempts at coiling as well as clipping.

Conclusion

A multidisciplinary decision is fundamental to decide whether an aneurysm is treated best by clipping or coiling. Future advances in endovascular techniques could change the overall management of unruptured aneurysm and more comparative studies involving unruptured aneurysms must be done to evaluate the pros and cons of clipping and coiling. However, despite major technical advances in imaging and in endovascular treatment of cerebral aneurysms, surgical clipping still is the most efficient treatment for unruptured MCA aneurysms at the beginning of the new millennium.

Acknowledgment

The authors want to thank Mrs Veronique Regli for the drawing.

References

1. Asari S, Ohmoto T (1993) Natural history and risk factors of unruptured cerebral aneurysms. Clin Neurol Neurosurg 95: 205–214

2. Chang HS, Kirino T (1995) Quantification of operative benefit for unruptured cerebral aneurysms: a theoretical approach. J Neurosurg 83: 413–420

3. Fernandez Zubillaga A, Gugliemi G, Viñuela F (1994) Endovascular occlusion of intracranial aneurysms with electrically detachable coils: correlation of aneurysm neck size and treatment results. AJNR 15: 815–820

4. Heiskanen O (1981) Risk of bleeding from unruptured aneurysms in cases with multiple intracranial aneurysms. J Neurosurg 55: 524–526

5. The International Study of Unruptured Intracranial Aneurysms Investigators (1998) Unruptured intracranial aneurysms – risk of rupture and risk of surgical intervention. N Engl J Med 339: 1725–1733

6. Jennett B, Bond M (1975) Assessment of outcome after severe brain damage. A practical scale. Lancet 1: 480–484

7. Juvela S, Porras M, Heiskanen O (1993) Natural history of unruptured intracranial aneurysms: a long-term follow-up study. J Neurosurg 79: 174–182

8. Khanna RK, Malik GM, Qureshi N (1996) Predicting outcome following surgical treatment of unruptured intracranial aneurysms: a proposed grading system. J Neurosurg 84: 49–54

9. King JT Jr, Berlin JA, Flamm ES (1994) Morbidity and mortality from elective surgery for asymptomatic, unruptured intracranial aneurysms: a meta-analysis. J Neurosurg 81: 837–842

10. King JT Jr, Glick HA, Mason TJ *et al* (1995) Elective surgery for asymptomatic, unruptured intracranial aneurysms: a cost-effectiveness analysis. J Neurosurg 83: 403–412

11. Kitanaka C, Tanaka JI, Kuwahara M *et al* (1994) Nonsurgical treatment of unruptured intracranial vertebral artery dissection with serial follow-up angiography. J Neurosurg 80: 667–674

12. Levy DI (1997) Embolization of wide-necked anterior communicating artery aneurysm: technical note. Neurosurgery 41: 979–982

13. Levy DI, Ku A (1997) Balloon-assisted coil placement in wide-necked aneurysms. Technical note. J Neurosurg 86: 724–727

14. Locksley HB (1966) Report on the Cooperative Study of intracranial aneurysms and subarachnoid hemorrhage. Section V, part II. Natural history of subarachnoid hemorrhage, intracranial aneurysms and arteriovenous malformations. Based on 6368 cases in the cooperative study. J Neurosurg 25: 321–368

15. Malisch TW, Gugliemi G, Viñuela F *et al* (1997) Intracranial aneurysms treated with Guglielmi detachable coil: midterm clinical results in a consecutive series of 100 patients. J Neurosurg 87: 176–183

16. Mericle RA, Wakhloo AK, Rodriguez R *et al* (1997) Temporary balloon protection as an adjunct to endosaccular coiling of wide-necked cerebral aneurysms: technical note. Neurosurgery 41: 975–978

17. Moret J, Cognard C, Weill A *et al* (1997) La technique de reconstruction dans le traitement des anévrismes intracrâniens à collet large. Résultats angiographiques et cliniques à long terms. A propos de 56 cas. J Neuroradiol 24: 30–44

18. Nakagawa T, Hashi K, (1994) The incidence and treatment of asymptomatic, unruptured cerebral aneurysms. J Neurosurg 80: 217–223

19. Obuchowski NA, Modic MT, Magdinec M (1995) Current implications for the efficacy of noninvasive screening for occult intracranial aneurysms in patients with a family history of aneurysms. J Neurosurg 83: 42–49

20. Orz Y, Kobayashi S, Osawa M *et al* (1997) Aneurysm size: a prognostic factor for rupture. Br J Neurosurg 11: 144–149

21. Regli L, Uske A, de Tribolet N (1999) Endovascular coil placement compared with surgical clipping for the treatment of unruptured middle cerebral artery aneurysm. J Neurosurg 90: 1025–1030

22. Rufenacht DA, Mandai S, Levrier O (1996) Endovascular treatment of intracranial aneurysms. AJNR 17: 1658–1660

23. Solomon RA, Fink ME, Pile-Spellman J (1994) Surgical management of unruptured intracranial aneurysms. J Neurosurg 80: 440–446

24. Viñuela F, Duckwiler G, Mawad M *et al* (1997) Guglielmi detachable coil embolization of acute intracranial aneurysm: perioperative anatomical and clinical outcome in 403 patients. J Neurosurg 86: 475–482

25. Wiebers DO, Torner JC, Meissner I (1992) Impact of unruptured intracranial aneurysms on public health in the United States. Stroke 23: 1416–1419

26. Wiebers DO, Whisnant JP, Sundt TM Jr *et al* (1987) The significance of unruptured intracranial saccular aneurysms. J Neurosurg 66: 23–29

27. Yasui N, Suzuki A, Nishimura H *et al* (1997) Long-term follow-up study of unruptured intracranial aneurysms. Neurosurgery 40: 1155–1160

Correspondence: Luca Regli, M.D., Médecin Associé, Department of Neurosurgery, Centre Hospitalier Vaudois, 1011 Lausanne, Switzerland.

Acta Neurochir (2002) [Suppl] 82: 47–49

Clinical Manifestations, Character of Aneurysms, and Surgical Results for Unruptured Cerebral Aneurysms Presenting with Ophthalmic Symptoms

A. Nishino, Y. Sakurai, H. Arai, S. Nishimura, S. Suzuki, and **H. Uenohara**

Department of Neurosurgery, Stroke Center, Sendai National Hospital, Sendai, Japan

Summary

Objects. Cases with unruptured cerebral aneurysms presenting with visual symptoms were investigated about their site, size, symptom, operative methods and results.

Material. Between 1984 and 1999, 8 cases were treated in Sendai National Hospital. One man and 7 women, mean age 66.4 years. Ophthalmic symptoms were as follows: diplopia in 6, visual acuity deterioration in 2, impaired visual field in 2 and ptosis in 3. Aneurysm location was IC cavernous in 3, IC ophthalmic in 3, ICPC in 1 and Acom in 1. Aneurysms of more than 25 mm numbered 6 cases.

Results. Operative methods and results were as follows: Direct clipping 3 cases, parent artery occlusion + EC/IC bypass 4 cases, Aneurysm trapping + EC/IC bypass 1 case. One patient who underwent direct clipping died following intraoperative complication. Of the remaining 7 cases, visual symptoms were improved in 4, remained unchanged in 2 cases, worsened in 1 case.

Conclusions. These results suggest that in cases with unruptured large or giant aneurysms presenting with ophthalmic symptoms, especially in IC cavernous or IC ophthalmic aneurysms, parent artery occlusion + EC/IC bypass is the safest operative procedure.

Keywords: Unruptured aneurysm; ophthalmic symptom; large aneurysm; EC/IC bypass; giant aneurysm.

Introduction

Unruptured cerebral aneurysms presenting ophthalmic symptoms are rare and tend to be large in size. Therefore, the strategies for the treatment of these aneurysms have not clearly been established.

In this study, we reviewed our surgical experiences with 8 unruptured cerebral aneurysm cases presenting with ophthalmic symptoms to investigate an optimal surgical method.

Clinical Material

Between 1984 and 1999, 8 patients with unruptured cerebral aneurysm presenting with ophthalmic symptoms were surgically treated at Sendai National Hospital. There were 7 women and 1 man with a mean age of 66.4 years. Ophthalmic symptoms were as follows: visual acuity deterioration in 2, impaired visual field in 3, diplopia in 6 and ptosis in 3. In 4 of the 8 patients, optic nerves were impaired and oculomotor or trochlear nerves were impaired in 6 patients. The aneurysms were located at the internal cerebral artery (IC) in 7 cases (IC cavernous 7, IC ophthalmic 3, IC PC 1) and 1 was at the anterior communicating artery. The size of aneuryms was between 20 and 25 mm in 2 cases and larger than 25 mm in 1 case.

Results

According to the site, location, and size of the aneurysms, our surgical procedures were as follows. IC ligation and extracranial-intracranial (EC/IC) bypass (STA-MCA 1, vein graft 1, radial artery graft 1) was performed in all 3 patients with IC cavernous aneurysms. Direct clipping was performed in 2 of 4 patients with IC ophthalmic or IC PC aneurysms, while IC ligation and EC/IC bypass (vein graft) was undergone in one patient, and aneurysm trapping and EC/IC bypass was performed also in one patient. In addition, direct clipping was performed in 1 patient with large Acom aneurysm.

Surgical complications are listed in Table 1. Two cases suffered from postoperative stroke, one was in the basal ganglia area followed by GOS 4 at discharge

Table 1. *Surgical Complication*

Site of AN	Surgery	Complications	Deficit	GOS
IC cavernous	IC ligation + vein graft bypass	infarction of basal ganglia	hemiparesis	4
IC ophthalmic	direct clipping	IC rupture	dead	
IC PC	direct clipping	infarction of internal capsule	hemiparesis	3

Table 2. *Change of the Ophthalmic Symptoms*

Site of AN	Surgery	Symptoms	Results
IC cavernous	IC ligation + bypass	rt. II,	unchanged
		rt. III, VI	improved
IC cavernous	IC ligation + bypass	rt. III	improved
IC cavernous	IC ligation + bypass	rt. VI	unchanged
IC ophthalmic	IC ligation + bypass	lt. III	improved
IC ophthalmic	AN trapping +	lt. III,	improved
	bypass	blt. II	lt; worsened
			rt; improved
IC ophthalmic	direct clipping	lt. II	(dead)
IC PC	direct clipping	rt. III	worsened
Acom	direct clipping	blt. II	improved

and the other was observed in the internal capsule area followed by GOS 3 at discharge. There was one death due to rupture of the internal carotid artery during inflation of the balloon catheter for temporally IC occlusion. Hence 2 out of the 3 patients treated with direct clipping had serious complications.

Changes of ophthalmic symptoms are summarized in Table 2. Three out of the 4 patients treated with parent artery occlusion and EC/IC bypass had a good outcome and improved their ophthalmic symptoms. One case treated with aneurysm trapping and EC/IC bypass had minimal defect of worsening ipsilateral visual acuity in spite of improving the contralateral visual acuity postoperatively.

Illustrative case

This 62-year-old woman was admitted with a 6-month history of decrease of her visual acuity (right: numerous digitorium, left: 0.03) with bitemporal hemianopsia. The left carotid angiography revealed an IC ophthalmic giant aneurysm (Fig. 1). Trapping of the aneurysm and EC/IC bypass using radial artery graft was performed. Postoperative angiography revealed enough collateral flow through the radial artery graft to the left MCA territory (Fig. 2). There is no CBF reduction at the left hemisphere on Tc PAO-SPECT.

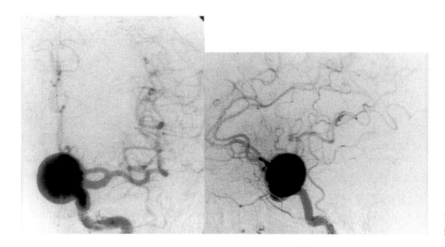

Fig. 1. The left carotid angiogram showing a giant IC ophthalmic aneurysm

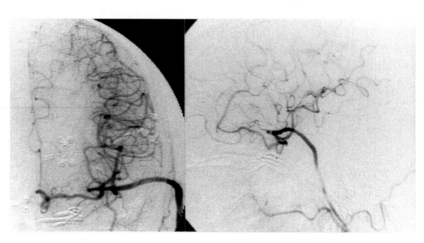

Fig. 2. Postoperative angiogram shows enough collateral flow through the radial artery graft to the left MCA territory with thrombotic obliteration of aneurysm

Discussion

Unruptured cerebral aneurysms presenting with ophthalmic symptoms are rare and tend to be large in size. Expanding cerebral aneurysm frequently injures the visual pathways and the ocular motor cranial nerves [1]. According to the literature, most unruptured aneurysms that produce neuro-ophthalmic signs arise from the junction of IC and Pcom arteries [2]. These aneurysms are reported to typically compress the third nerve in the subarachnoid space. However, in this study, unruptured aneurysms of the internal carotid artery induced 7 cases in the IC cavernous portion, 3 cases in the IC ophthalmic portion, IC PC in only 1 case. Since cases with headache were excluded from our series and the proximal and distal segments of the intracranial portion of IC compress the anterior visual pathways 5 out of the total 8 cases had visual acuity and/or visual field impairment.

The strategies for the treatment of these aneurysms seem to have not been established [3]. However, we suggest that in cases with unruptured large or giant aneurysms presenting ophthalmic symptoms, especially in IC cavernous or IC ophthalmic aneurysm cases, parent artery ligation and EC/IC bypass is the safest operative method. In cases requiring an aneurysm trapping procedure, gentle manipulation for the surrounding optic nerves is recommended.

References

1. Biousse V, Newman NJ (1999) Aneurysms and Subarachnoid hemorrhage. Neursurg Clin N Am 10: 631–651
2. Kasner SE, Liu GT, Galetta SL (1997) Neuro-ophthalmologic aspects of aneurysms. Neuroimaging Clin N Am 7: 679–692
3. Drake CG, Peerless SJ, Ferguson GG (1994) Hunterian proximal arterial occlusion for giant aneurysms of the carotid circulation. J Neurosurg 81: 656–665

Correspondence: Akiko Nishino, Department of Neurosurgery, Sendai National Hospital Address: 2-8-8, Miyagino, Miyagino-ku, Sendai, Japan.

Acta Neurochir (2002) [Suppl] 82: 51–54

Clinical Outcome after Surgery of Intracranial Unruptured Aneurysms: Results of a Series Between 1991 and 2001

R. G. Hempelmann, H. Barth, R. Buhl, and **H. M. Mehdorn**

Department of Neurosurgery, University of Kiel, Kiel, Germany

Summary

The clinical results of surgery for unruptured aneurysms in the Neurosurgical Department of Kiel were analyzed to further discuss whether an operative treatment can be advised.

Between 1991 and 2001, 54 unruptured aneurysms in 45 patients were operated in our department.

No complications occurred in 38 patients; transient complications (slight aphasia, hemiparesis, psychiatric disorders) in 4 patients; postoperative seizures in one, epidural haematoma with the need of re-operation in one, and infection in another patient. At the time of discharge, GOS was 5 in 33 patients, 4 in 12 patients. But the slight disabilities were due to the aneurysm operation only in two patients, in the other 10 patients they were caused by pre-existing concomitant diseases. The Rankin-Scale after at least 6 months was 1 (no disability) in 31 patients (37 patients investigated); 2 (slight disability) in 5, and 3 (moderate disability) in one patient. In only one of these patients, the slight disability was caused by the aneurysm operation. During a telephone interview performed between 6 months and 7 years after the operation, all patients except two (31 patients investigated) gave a positive answer to the question, whether, in case of diagnosis of an aneurysm, they would undergo an operation again.

Regarding our results, we still advocate treatment of unruptured aneuryms in patients who are in stable clinical conditions, especially in young patients and in patients with unique aneurysm configurations and aneurysm sizes approaching 10 mm.

Keywords: Unruptured intracranial aneurysms; operative treatment; outcome; telephone interview.

Introduction

The recommendations for the treatment of unruptured intracranial aneurysms have been controversial during the last years. The most recent large meta-analysis involving 2460 patients demonstrated a morbidity rate of 10.9% and a mortality rate of 2.6% after surgery for unruptured aneurysms [7]. The ISUIA researchers [4] presented a comprehensive retrospective as well as prospective investigation on the risk of rupture versus the risk of surgical treatment of un-

ruptured aneurysms, encompassing a total of 2621 patients. The mortality rates of surgical interventions were 3.8% at 1 year for patients without a history of prior subarachnoid haemorrhage (SAH), and 1% at 1 year for those with a previous SAH owing to a different aneurysm. The neurological disability rates including the cognitive disability rates at 1 year were 12% for both patient groups. The paper showed, in contrast to previous reports [1, 5, 6, 9, 10], that the cumulative risk of rupture was low, namely less than 0.05% per year, when no history of SAH from a different aneurysm existed, whereas the risk was about 11 times higher in patients who underwent a successful operation on a ruptured aneurysm previously.

The ISUIA study examined the functional outcome after aneurysm operation by means of validated scales. An important question, as mentioned by Bederson *et al.* [2], is the quality of life living with the diagnosis of an incidental or unruptured aneurysm. Between 1991 and 2001, 45 patients harbouring 54 unruptured aneurysms were operated in our department. We assessed the outcome of these patients using the Telephone Interview for Cognitive Status [3] as well as the Rankin scale [8], according to the procedure in the ISUIA study. The patients were asked, whether they would undergo the operation again including the experienced postoperative course and putative complications.

Methods

All patients operated on an unruptured aneurysm between January 1991 and January 2001 were included, whether the aneurysm was symptomatic (cranial nerve palsy) or not. The patient's data (i.e. the history, the symptoms, concomitant diseases, localisation and size of aneurysm, the type of operation (clipping or wrapping), the complications and the GOS score, were evaluated and digitised prospectively in all of our intensive care patients. These digitised data have been completed and compared with data, retrospectively evaluated from the patient's records and documents.

The long term-outcome was assessed by the Telephone Interview for Cognitive Status [3]. Furthermore, the Rankin scale [8] was ascertained, and the patients were asked, whether they suffered from residual symptoms such as headache, sleeplessness, dizziness, irritation, fatigue, disturbances of concentration, vision, speech or motion, seizures, nausea or other disturbances of their physical condition.

The telephone interview was performed between 0.5 and 7 years after discharge of the patients. In 2 patients, the interview was not performed, because they had been operated on recently.

Results

45 patients harbouring 54 aneurysms were treated between 1991 and the beginning of 2001 in the Department of Neurosurgery in Kiel, the characteristics of the patients are shown in Table 1. The mean age was 51 years (12–75 years). Approximately two thirds of the patients were women, seven patients underwent operative interventions on multiple aneurysms, including the two patients who suffered from arteriovenous malformations (AVM). Only one of our patients had a symptomatic aneurysm, in three patients who had successfully been operated on a ruptured aneurysm previously, a second, unruptured aneurysm was diagnosed and operatively clipped later on. All other aneurysms were incidental aneurysms, found on the occasion of diagnostic procedures due to different symptoms or diseases. Thus, excluding the aneurysms seen in patients with AVM, 39 patients had incidental aneurysms. Of these patients, 26 had aneurysms smaller than 10 mm, where in consideration of the low risk of haemorrhage reported in the ISUIA, observation rather than operation is recommended. Three patients had giant aneurysms.

Three aneurysms were treated by wrapping (including one giant aneurysm), two aneuryms by resection and reconstruction of the vessel's wall or by end-to-side-anastomosis, one aneurysm (anterior communicating artery) by trapping.

Except one aneurysm of the posterior communicating artery, all aneurysms belonged to the anterior circulation (middle cerebral artery: 21, internal carotid artery: 16, anterior communicating artery: 12, anterior cerebral artery: 4).

Most of the incidental aneurysms were found by radiological clarification of headache or migraine, benign intracranial tumours, ischemic attacks or carotid

Table 1. *Pre-Operative Characteristics*

Patient and aneurysm characteristics	Number
Number of patients	45
Females	31
Males	14
Mean Age (years)	51
Range (years)	12–75
Total number of aneurysms	54
Patients with a single aneurysm	38
Patients with multiple aneurysms	7
Incidental aneurysms	46
AVM with 2 aneurysms (No. of patients)	2
Symptomatic aneurysms	1
Asymptomatic aneurysms after SAH	3
Location of aneurysms (numbers)	
Middle cerebral artery	21
Internal carotid artery	16
Anterior communicating artery	12
Anterior cerebral artery	4
Posterior communicating artery	1
Size of largest aneurysm (numbers)	
Small (<8 mm)	11
Approaching 10 mm	15
10–20 mm	16
>20 mm	3
Conditions leading to aneurysm diagnosis	
Headache or migraine	11
Benign intracranial tumour	8
Carotid stenosis	7
Syncopes of unknown etiology	3
Psychiatric disorders	2
Arteriovenous malformations	2
Others (normal pressure hydrocephalus, endocrine orbitopathy, neuritis of optic nerve, seizure, diagnostics due to carcinoma, to cardiac disease, or to hyperthyroidism, trauma)	8
Short-termed palsy of third nerve	1
SAH due to different aneurysm	3

artery stenosis and syncopes of unknown etiology (31 patients, see also Table 1).

Postoperative complications occurred in 7 patients, in four of these patients, the problems were transient (aphasia, seizures, or psychiatric disorders in two cases) and subsided even before discharge from the hospital. One patient had a permanent, operation-induced slight hemiparesis and aphasia, that did not substantially disturb the patient's daily life. One female patient had a severe infection with meningitis and osteomyelitis that warranted further operative therapy and a long stay in the clinic. Another female patient suffered from postoperative epidural haematoma due to coagulation disorders that were not diagnosed pre-operatively, and had to be re-operated. This patient completely recovered afterwards.

Table 2. *Complications and Outcome Data*

Complications	number of patients	2 months later
No complication	38	
Slight hemiparesis and aphasia	1	complete recovery
Transient aphasia	1	complete recovery
Postoperative seizures	1	anticonvulsive therapy
Re-bleeding and re-operation	1	complete recovery
Meningitis and osteomyelitis	1	moderate disability
Transient psychiatric disorder	2	complete recovery
GOS score at discharge	*number of patients*	
5	33 (73%)	
4	12 (27%)	
due to:		
Aneurysm operation	2	
Intracranial tumour operation	5	
Infarct owing to carotid stenosis	1	
Carotid endarterectomy	1	
AVM operation	1	
Rankin-Scale after at least 6 months (total: 37 patients)		
1 (no disability)	*31 (84%)*	
2 (slight disability)	*5 (14%)*	
due to:		
Aneurysm operation	1	
Intracranial tumour	1	
Carotid stenosis	1	
Cardiac disease	1	
Previous SAH	1	
3 (moderate disability)	*1 (2%)*	
due to intracranial tumour	1	
Telephone interview for cognitive status (total: 29 patients)		
>30 (normal)	24 (83%)	
<30 (cognitive disability)	5 (17%)	
putatively due to:		
Aneurysm operation	2	
Intracranial tumour	3	

The GCS score at time of discharge amounted to 5 in 33 patients who did not suffer from complications and no considerable complaints at the end of their stay in hospital. In 12 patients, the GCS score was 4, but only in 2 patients this was explained by an operation-related clinical deterioration. The other patients were slightly handicapped owing to the other diseases that led to the diagnosis of the incidental aneurysms, i.e. benign intracranial tumours or ischemic deficits. Altogether, 7 patients endured an operation-induced considerable clinical worsening, that was still present in 2 patients at the time of discharge (with infection and with post-operative seizures and necessary anticonvulsive therapy).

Three patients died during the following years due to operation-unrelated reasons (intracranial tumour, cardiac disease, lung carcinoma).

The Rankin-Scale was evaluated by clinical follow-up examinations more than six months after the operation or by the telephone interview. It amounted to 1 (no disability) in 31 patients (84%) from 37 investigated and 2 (slight disability) in 5 patients (14%), but only in 1 patient this was due to the aneurysm treatment. It amounted to 3 (moderate disability) in 1 patient (due to intracranial tumour operation).

The telephone interview was performed with 31 patients. Two of these patients answered to questions concerning their physical condition, but refused to answer to the Telephone Interview for Cognitive Status. Three patients had died because of aneurysm-unrelated reasons. Two patients were not phoned because of a recent operation. Nine patients were lost to follow-up.

The Telephone Interview for Cognitive Status demonstrated normal values in 24 patients (83%) from 29 patients questioned. In 5 patients (17%) the index was below 31 points, indicating cognitive disability. Putatively, this was caused by the aneurysm operation in 2 patients, and by intracranial tumour in 3 patients.

One patient would not undergo the operation again because of the re-bleeding, though she had no residual symptoms. One patient did not feel able to give a certain answer because of pre-existing headache that was aggravated after the operation. All other patients [27] including the woman suffering from meningitis and osteomyelitis gave a clear positive answer to the question whether they would decide to undergo the operation again, including the experienced postoperative course, in case of the diagnosis of an aneurysm. The patients prefered to be operated rather than to live with the knowledge of the existence of an untreated intracranial aneurysm.

Discussion

The meta-analyses and studies of the recent years, especially the ISUIA study encompassing more than 2600 patients, led to new recommendations for the management of patients with unruptured intracranial aneurysms [2, 4]. The ISUIA study revealed that the natural course of unruptured aneurysms was substantially different between patients with previous subarachnoid haemorrhage (SAH) due to a different, successfully clipped aneurysm and those who did not experience previous SAH. Another important aspect in the natural history of unruptured aneurysms is the aneurysm size. The study showed, that the likelihood of rupture of an aneurysm less than 10 mm in diameter was less than 0.05% per year in patients with no previous SAH due to a different aneurysm. These data contrasted previous findings with a higher cumulative rupture rate [1, 5, 6, 9, 10]. They led to the recommendations, that those patients with incidental small aneurysms and without a previous SAH history should rather be observed than treated. Exceptions may be considerably younger patients, patients with a positive familiy history, and aneurysms with unique configurations [2]. Another important argument is the patient's personal opinion whether she or he can bear the knowledge of harbouring an intracranial aneurysm or not.

During the last ten years, 54 unruptured aneurysms in 45 patients have been operated in our department. After publication of the ISUIA study, we reviewed the data and documents of the patients and performed telephone interviews to get actual information about the further course:

In the 45 patients, two major complications occurred. The female patient suffering from meningitis and osteomyelitis did not completely recover from the operation (Rankin 2), but would undergo an aneurysm intervention again. The second severe complication was an epidural hematoma after combined tumour and aneurysm operation. The patient was reoperated and recovered completely, but would not undergo an operation again. The other postoperative complications were transient and subsided during the following weeks except seizures in one female patient who had to be treated with anticonvulsive medication. All other slight and moderate disabilities were due to concomitant diseases or to operations of intracranial tumours, but not related to the aneurysm treatment.

With only two exceptions all patients, including the woman with the worst complications (infection), confirmed that they would undergo an operation again in the case of harbouring an intracranial aneurysm.

Hence, the permanent morbidity of the operations was low, and, in our opinion, even the observed complications do not convincingly argue against the operative treatment.

We operated 26 patients with an aneurysm size less than 10 mm and no history of a previous SAH, i.e. patients with a reportedly low risk of haemorrhage [4]. Of course, the patients must be thoroughly informed about the apparently low risk of rupture and the conceivable risks of the operation. But concerning our operative results, we still advocate the neurosurgical intervention, especially in young patients and in clinically stable patients with unique aneurysm configurations or aneurysm diameters approaching 10 mm.

References

1. Asari S, Ohmoto T (1993) Natural history and risk factors of unruptured cerebral aneurysms. Clin Neurol Neurosurg 95: 205–214
2. Bederson JB, Awad IA, Wiebers DO *et al* (2000) Recommendations for the management of patients with unruptured intracranial aneurysms. Circulation 102: 2300–2308
3. Brandt J, Spencer M, Folstein M (1988) Telephone Interview for Cognitive Status. Neuropsychiatr Neuropsychol Behav Neurol 1: 111–117
4. ISUIA investigators (1998) Unruptured intracranial aneurysms: risks of rupture and risks of surgical intervention. N Engl J Med 339: 1725–1733
5. Jane JA, Kassell NF, Torner JC *et al* (1985) The natural history of aneurysms and AVMs. J Neurosurg 62: 321–323
6. Locksley HB (1966) Natural history of subarachnoid hemorrhage, intracranial aneurysms and arteriovenous malformations. J Neurosurg 25: 321–368
7. Raaymakers TW, Rinkel GJ, Limburg M *et al* (1998) Mortality and morbidity of surgery for unruptured intracranial aneurysms: a meta-analysis. Stroke 29: 1531–1538
8. Rankin J (1957) Cerebral vascular accidents in patients over age 60. II. Prognosis. Scott Med J 2: 200–215
9. Yasui N, Magarisawa S, Suzuki A *et al* (1996) Subarachnoid hemorrhage caused by previously diagnosed, previously unruptured intracranial aneurysms: a retrospective analysis of 25 cases. Neurosurgery 39: 1096–1100
10. Yasui N, Suzuki A, Nishimura H *et al* (1997) Long-term follow-up study of unruptured intracranial aneurysms. Neurosurgery 40: 1155–1159

Correspondence: R. G. Hempelmann, Neurochirurgische Universitätsklinik Kiel, Weimarer Strasse 8, D-24106 Kiel, Germany.

Acta Neurochir (2002) [Suppl] 82: 55–58
© Springer-Verlag 2002

Radiation-Induced Cerebral Aneurysm Successfully Treated with Endovascular Coil Embolization

N. Murakami, T. Tsukahara, H. Toda, O. Kawakami, and T. Hatano

Department of Neurosurgery and Clinical Research Unit, Kyoto National Hospital, Kyoto, Japan

Summary

In a 30-year-old male, multiple cerebral aneurysms developed 19 years after receiving 60 Gy of irradiation for craniophariginoma. Angiogram revealed right IC-PC and upper basilar trunk aneurysms in addition to atherosclerotic change. The right IC-PC aneurysm was wrapped and the basilar trunk aneurysm located between the origins of SCA and AICA was treated by endovascular coil embolization. The packing of the aneurysm was complete, but stenosis of the basilar artery appeared. The patient was discharged uneventfully and follow-up angiogram 6 months later demonstrated that the aneurysm had disappeared and the patency of the basilar artery had been preserved. Radiation-induced intracranial vasculopathy is a well-recognized phenomenon, but aneurysm formation is less common than arterial occlusive lesion. However, the mortality rate after bleeding is so high that immediate diagnosis and treatment by direct surgery or coil embolization are necessary.

Keywords: Radiation; cerebral aneurysm; embolization; Guglielmi detachable coils.

Introduction

Radiation-induced vasculopathy is now well accepted and stenosis, occlusion, and moyamoya vascular changes are often described, but intracranial aneurysm formation is rare. Only 13 cases have previously been reported [1–6, 9, 10] and 9 of 13 patients developed subarachnoid hemorrhage. Six of these 9 patients died representing a mortality rate of 67%, and successful treatment was very difficult. We demonstrate a case in which the developing aneurysm after radiation therapy was successfully treated with endovascular coil embolization.

Case Report

A 30-year-old male received 60 Gy of radiation to a suprasellar tumor in 1981 and was thereafter medicated for panhypopituitarism and hyperlipidemia sec-

ondary to hypothyroidism. A recurrent tumor was partially removed 10 years later and the histological diagnosis was craniopharigioma. Postoperative sequential brain magnetic resonance imaging (MRI) showed that the residual tumor had not changed in size for 9 years, but brain MRI obtained in 2000 showed that cystic lesions had appeared in the bilateral basal ganglia and the right temporal lobe. To verify the diagnosis of the cystic lesions, angiography was performed and the right IC-PC and upper basilar trunk aneurysms were demonstrated in addition to several stenoses in the neighboring arteries (Fig. 1). On April 4, 2000, wrapping of the right IC-PC aneurysm and biopsy of the cystic lesion in the right temporal lobe were performed. The biopsy specimens showed ischemic change that might be due to the previous radiation therapy. The basilar trunk aneurysm was located between the origins of SCA and AICA, projecting posteriorly with a size of 5 mm in diameter. Therefore, direct surgery for the aneurysm was thought to be very difficult and endovascular coil embolization was performed on June 2, 2000. Under general anesthesia with intravenous heparin administration, an 8F guiding catheter was placed in the right vertebral artery via the right femoral artery. Tracker 38 microcatheter (Boston Scientific Co., USA) introduced in the basilar artery and then a second Excelsior microcatheter (Boston Scientific Co., USA) was placed into the aneurysm with coaxial technique. Six Guglielmi electrodetachable coils (GDCs) (Boston Scientific Co., USA) consisting of a 4 mm-helix × 8 cm length, two 3 mm-helix × 8 cm length, two 2 mm helix × 8 cm length and a 2 mm helix × 6 cm length coils were introduced into the aneurysm. The packing of the aneurysm was complete, but stenosis of the basilar artery appeared

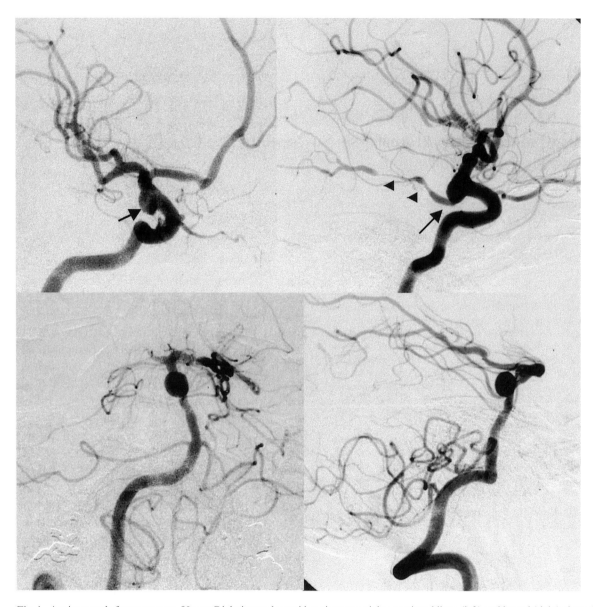

Fig. 1. Angiograms before treatment. Upper: Right internal carotid angiograms, right anterior oblique (left) and lateral (right) views showing right IC-PC aneurysm situated directly on the origin of right posterior communicating artery (arrows). The proximal segment of right posterior cerebral artery appears stenotic (arrowheads). Lower: Right vertebral angiograms, anteroposterior (left) and lateral (right) views, showing basilar trunk aneurysm located between the origins of SCA and AICA, projecting posteriorly

due to the broad neck. After coil embolization, the patient received antiplatelet therapy and was discharged uneventfully. Follow-up angiogram obtained 6 months later demonstrated that the aneurysm was completely embolized and the patency of the basilar artery was preserved (Fig. 2).

Discussion

In 1984, Azzarelli *et al.* first reported an intracranial aneurysm following radiation therapy for suprasel-

lar germinoma [1] but reports of radiation-induced aneurysms are rare, only 13 cases have previously been published [1–6, 9, 10]. These reports showed that the rupture and mortality rate of untreated radiation-induced aneurysms were so high that immediate diagnosis and treatment are thought to be important. Regarding diagnosis, MR angiography can be used to investigate aneurysm as well as atherosclerosis of intracranial major artery noninvasively. It has been shown that risk factors in the pathogenesis of radiation-induced arteriosclerosis are hyperlipidemia [7],

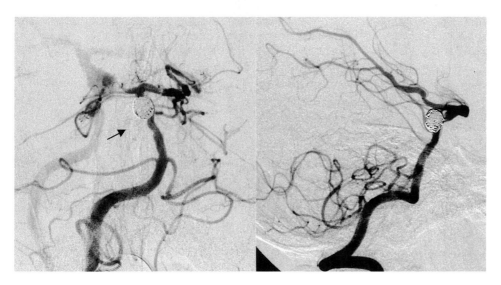

Fig. 2. Angiograms 6 months after treatment. Right vertebral angiograms, anteroposterior (left) and lateral (right) views show complete embolization of basilar trunk aneurysm with parent artery stenosis

hypothyroidism and early age [11], so sequential follow-up of vascular pathology should be performed in patients with some of these risk factors who have received radiation therapy for benign intracranial tumor. However, special attention must be paid to the treatment of radiation-induced aneurysms, because these aneurysms differ from congenital saccular aneurysms by virtue of shape and location. For example, radiation-induced aneurysms often arise directly from a segment of major artery and are associated with atherosclerotic change in the neighboring arteries, situated in the radiation field. So, radiation-induced aneurysms often have a broad neck and arterial branches from the aneurysmal wall, and it is difficult to perform direct clipping. In our case, the right IC-PC aneurysm had a broad neck with atherosclerotic change of the parent artery and the posterior communicating artery arose from the aneurysmal wall, so we decided that clipping of the aneurysm was impossible and hence performed wrapping of the aneurysm. Then, we chose endovascular treatment for the basilar trunk aneurysm because of the location. Previously in one patient, endovascular coil embolization was attempted, but fatal bleeding followed 2 weeks later [6]. Our case is the first reported successful treatment of a radiation-induced aneurysm using endovascular coil embolization. Recently, interventional neuroradiology has progressed remarkably and coil embolization of cerebral aneurysms is performed with low mortality and morbidity [8]. Therefore, if a radiation-induced aneurysm is diagnosed in a region inaccessible for direct surgery, the endovascular treatment is thought to be one of the therapeutic choices.

References

1. Azzarelli B, Moore J, Gilmor R, Muller L, Edwards M, Mealer J (1984) Multiple fusiform intracranial aneurysms following curative radiation therapy for suprasellar germinoma. J Neurosurg 61: 1141–1145
2. Benson PJ, Sung JH (1989) Cerebral aneurysms following radiotherapy for medulloblastoma. J Neurosurg 70: 545–550
3. Casey ATH, Marsh HT, Uttley D (1993) Short report. Intracranial aneurysm formation following radiotherapy. Br J Neurosurg 7: 575–579
4. Gomori JM, Levy P, Weshler Z (1987) Radiation-induced aneurysm of the basilar artery. A case report. Angiology 38: 147–150
5. Jensen FK, Wagner A (1997) Intracranial aneurysm following radiation therapy for medulloblastoma. A case report and review of the literature. Acta Radiol 38: 37–42
6. John DG, Porter MJ, Van Hasselt CA, Med M (1993) Clinical records. Beware of bleeding from the ear. J Laryngol Otol 107: 137–139
7. Kirkpatrick JB (1967) Pathogenesis of foam cell lesions in irradiated arteries. Am J Pathol 50: 291–300
8. Malish TW, Guglielmi G, Venuela F, Duckwiler G, Gobin YP, Martin NA, Frazee JG (1997) Intracranial aneurysms treated with the Guglielmi detachable coil: mid-term clinical results in a consecutive series of 100 patients. J Neurosurg 87: 176–183
9. Nishi T, Matsukado Y, Kodama T, Hiraki T (1987) Multiple intracranial aneurysms following radiation therapy for pituitary adenoma. Neurol Med Chir 27: 224–228
10. Scodary DJ, Tew JM, Thomas GM, Tomsick T, Liwnicz BH (1990) Radiation-induced cerebral aneurysms. Acta Neurochi (Wien) 102: 141–144

11. Smith C, Loewenthal LA (1950) A study of elastic arteries in ir-
    radiated mice of different ages. Proc Soc Exp Biol Med 75: 859–
    861

Correspondence: Nobukuni Murakami, Department of Neurosurgery and Clinical Research Unit, Kyoto National Hospital, 1-1,
Mukaihata-cho, Fushimi-ku, Kyoto 612-8555, Japan.

Part II: Treatment of Subarachnoid Haemorrhage and General Considerations

Acta Neurochir (2002) [Suppl] 82: 61–64

Surgery and Outcome for Aneurysmal Subarachnoid Hemorrhage in Elderly Patients

M. O. Pinsker, W. Gerstner, S. Wolf, H. A. Trost, and **C. B. Lumenta**

Department of Neurosurgery, Academic Hospital Munich-Bogenhausen, Munich, Germany

Summary

Objective. The goal was to report treatment results of elderly patients (over 70 years) who underwent clipping of aneurysms after subarachnoid hemorrhage (SAH).

Material and Methods. From 1994 to 2000 41/284 (14%) patients older than 70 years were operated on aneurysmal SAH in our department. Localization of ruptured aneurysm was anterior communicating artery (n = 14), middle cerebral artery (n = 14), internal carotid artery (n = 6), anterior cerebral artery (n = 2), pericallosal artery (n = 1) and multiple in 4 patients. We used the Hunt and Hess classification for initial grading and the Glasgow Outcome Score at day 30 after surgery.

Results. Patients with HH 1–3 had a low mortality (1/18, 6%), whereas 9 of 23 patients (39%) with HH 4–5 deceased within 30 days after surgery. Overall mortality was 24.5% (10/41) at 30 days after surgery. Most patients (n = 32) underwent early surgery (within 72 hours). Shunt dependent hydrocephalus developed in 15 patients (37%). The outcome was better in patients graded HH 1–3, in those without serious atherosclerotic changes in angiography, and in AcoA and ICA localization compared to MCA.

Conclusion. Advanced age does not preclude successful surgery for ruptured aneurysm. Most important factor for outcome was a good initial clinical status, though the majority of our patients presented with poor grades. Early surgical clipping and postoperative intensive care can attain a favorable outcome in a significant percentage of elderly patients.

Keywords: Subarachnoid hemorrhage; age; outcome.

Introduction

Case-fatality rates after subarachnoid hemorrhage have decreased during the last three decades [6]. Explanations for this are improvements in diagnostic, surgical and intensive care management techniques. Combined with a growing elderly population, the number of operations for ruptured intracranial aneurysms also increased [18]. Recent studies showed that due to improving results, especially in elderly patients [8, 10] a more aggressive approach seems to be justified. On the other hand, the reported mortality of elderly patients with ruptured aneurysms is up to 45% [3] and the overall outcome much worse compared to younger patients [11, 12, 13] due to the primary brain damage, due to the poorer clinical status on admission and due to associated preexisting medical conditions of these patients.

To evaluate whether surgery is justified by the outcome in this patient group, we retrospectively analyzed our experiences with surgery on 41 elderly patients with aneurysmal subarachnoid hemorrhage, considering the computerized tomography (CT) findings, neurological grade on admission, site of ruptured aneurysms, vascular status on angiography and outcome.

Material and Methods

We reviewed patient files, operating charts, computed tomography (CT) scans and angiography series of 41 patients older than 70 years of age who underwent surgical clipping of ruptured cerebral aneurysms from January 1994 to December 2000. Patients' age ranged from 70 years to 79 years, with a median of 72 years. Male to female ratio was 11:30. As published previously [15] we found the following risk factors for subarachnoid hemorrhage in our patients: arterial hypertonus in 14 patients; cardiovascular diseases, e.g. coronary heart disease, in 12 patients, and diabetes mellitus in 12 patients. Six patients, median age was 76 years, with subarachnoid hemorrhage on CT-scans were excluded from this study, because they did not undergo surgery due to a very poor clinical status at the time of admission to our department (4 patients) or due to an advanced carcinoma (2 patients). All of them died within four days after the hemorrhage.

All patients underwent angiography preoperatively, in 8 cases only the side highly suspective for aneurysm localization was investigated in order to save time. To rule out another aneurysm in these patients we performed CT-angiography or MR-angiography after clinical recovery. Most common were aneurysms of the anterior communicating artery (AcoA) and the middle cerebral artery (MCA) in 14/41 patients (34%) each. Aneurysms in the internal carotid ar-

Table 1. *Outcome of all Patients at Day 30 after Surgery*

	Number of patients	%
GOS 5 (good recovery)	10	24.5
GOS 4 (moderate deficit)	7	17
GOS 3 (severe deficit)	9	22
GOS 2 (vegetative state)	5	12
GOS 1 (dead)	10	24.5

Table 2. *Outcome of Poor Grade Patients with Hunt/Hess Grade 4 and 5 at Day 30 after Surgery*

	HH 4	HH 5
GOS 5	0	0
GOS 4	4 (27%)	0
GOS 3	5 (33%)	1 (12.5%)
GOS 2	3 (20%)	1 (12.5%)
GOS 1	3 (20%)	6 (75%)
Total	15	8

Table 3. *Outcome at Day 30 after Surgery Related to Localization of Aneurysms*

	AcoA	MCA	ACA	ICA	A2	Multiple
GOS 5	4	1	2	1	0	0
GOS 4	3	2	2	0	0	1
GOS 3	3	4	1	0	1	2
GOS 2	2	1	1	0	0	1
GOS 1	2	6	0	1	0	0
Total	14	14	6	2	1	4

tery were located in 6 patients (15%), followed by two aneurysms in the anterior cerebral artery (5%), and one aneurysm in the A2-segment. Four of 41 patients (10%) had more than one aneurysm.

We divided the patients into two groups based on the results of angiography: those with a "poor" vascular status (n = 7, 17%), (extensive atherosclerotic changes compared to the average angiography in this age group or a previous history of a cerebrovascular accident), and those with "normal" vascular status (n = 34, 83%).

Clinical grading was done according to the Hunt and Hess classification of subarachnoid hemorrhage [7] and using the Fisher scale for CT-findings [4].

Results

Three patients out of 41 (7%) were graded HH 1, 10/41 (24.5%) were HH 2, 5/41 (12%) patients were HH 3, 15/41 patients (37%) were HH 4 and 8/41 patients (19.5%) were HH 5. Based on CT-scanning there were 11 patients (27%) Fisher grade 2, 8 patients (19%) Fisher grade 3 and 22 patients (54%) Fisher grade 4.

Surgery was done within 72 hours (so-called early surgery) in 32 cases (78%), and after 10 days in nine patients (22%), so called late-surgery. Reasons for late surgery were due to a transfer to our department after day 3 after the hemorrhage or due to initial refusal of the patients.

An external ventricular drainage due to hydrocephalus was implanted perioperatively in 28 patients (68%). Fifteen (37% of all) of them developed a shunt-dependent hydrocephalus demanding ventriculo-peritoneal shunt implantation within 12 days (median) after initial hemorrhage.

There was no rebleeding after surgery, cerebral infarctions in 11 patients and vasospasm detected by transcranial doppler sonography in 14 patients. Three patients underwent a percutaneous tracheostomy due to a long-term ventilation.

The patient outcome was graded upon the Glasgow Outcome Scale (GOS) (see Table 1 for details).

Related to the initial grading 10/18 (56%) patients out of the Hunt/Hess 1–3 group had an excellent outcome (GOS 5), with only one deceased patient in this group (5% mortality). In the Hunt/Hess 4–5 group 9 of 23 patients (40%) had died 30 days after surgery.

Further splitting of the outcome related to initial clinical condition showed very poor outcome of HH 5 patients. Six of eight patients graded HH 5 were dead on day 30 after surgery, one patient was vegetative, and one patient had a severe neurological deficit (GOS 3). Nevertheless, four patients graded HH 4 had an acceptable outcome (GOS 4), but five had a severe deficit, 3 remained vegetative and 3 patients died. The overall mortality on day 30 after surgery was 24.5%.

Mortality of patients with a so-called "poor" vascular status (3/7 patients, 43%) was twice of those with "normal" vascular status (7/34 patients, 21%). On the other hand, only one patient with "poor" vascular status had vasospasm in TCD. The outcome related to aneurysm location is shown in detail in Table 3.

Although the numbers are too small for statistical analysis, the outcome seemed to be better in patients with aneurysms in the AcoA or in the ICA compared to patients with aneurysms in the MCA.

Discussion

The number and the proportion of elderly people in industrial countries has increased in the last years and will increase in the future [5, 18]. Additionally the incidence of ruptured cerebral aneurysms is higher in older patients compared to younger ones. In the Framingham study the annual incidence of SAH per

100.000 population increased from 15 in the 30- to 59 year-old group to 78 in the 70- to 88-year-old group [17]. Others, e.g. Fridriksson *et al.* [5], reported a much lower annual incidence of 16 per 100.000 population per year for patients older than 70 years. Broderick *et al.* [2] reported an overall annual incidence of only six per 100.000 population for SAH.

Due to improvements in management strategies combined with a growing proportion of elderly people, the number of operated elderly patients with ruptured cerebral aneurysms has increased [18]. Recent studies [11, 12, 13] reported a percentage from 23- to 26% of patients above 60 years of age. In our study, 14% of our SAH patients were older than 70 years. The management of cerebral aneurysms in this group of patients is becoming an increasingly important issue in neurosurgical centres dealing with those patients.

Several factors contributing to an unfavorable outcome after aneurysmal rupture in elderly patients have been proposed [13, 15], such as poor neurological grade on admission, cerebral vasospasm, and pre-existing medical conditions such as hypertension, diabetes mellitus, cardiopulmonary and cerebrovascular disease. Overall outcome is largely determined by initial hemorrhage, by intracranial hypertension and by cerebral infarction [14].

More than half of our patients were in a bad clinical condition on admission, Hunt/Hess grade 4 or 5. Twenty-two patients had a CT-scan graded a Fisher 4, i.e. with intracerebral or intraventricular clot.

The larger amount of subarachnoid blood can be explained by the parenchymal atrophy due to degenerative processes in the elderly. Additionally the presence of elevated blood pressure is related to the severity of SAH [13].

Bailes *et al.* [1] concluded from their results with poor-grade aneurysm patients, that an immediate ventriculostomy should be performed, since increased ICP can be present, even in cases without ventriculomegaly. We have performed a ventriculostomy only in patients presenting with signs of hydrocephalus or hematocephalus (n = 28, 68%). Fifteen of them (37%) developed a shunt-dependent hydrocephalus, which was performed ventriculo-peritoneally in all cases, in median 12 days after the initial hemorrhage. Compared to the complete collective (284 patients, operated on from 1994 to 2000), shunt-dependency was higher (37% versus 18%) and implantation was performed earlier (12 days versus 19 days). This might be due to the high incidence of severe SAH in the

elderly group (Fisher grade 4), but another reason might be the urge to get them earlier independent of external catheters due to the risk of infections, and consequently earlier discharge from intensive care units.

We found a better outcome in patients without extensive atherosclerotic changes in the angiography and/or without the history of cerebrovascular accidents (CVA) compared to those who presented with large plaques, elongations or a history of cerebrovascular disease. The ability to compensate the physiological reduction in cerebral blood flow during normal aging [16] might be passed in these patients.

According to the results of the International Cooperative Study Group on the timing of aneurysm surgery [11, 12] we advocate the early surgery of ruptured aneurysms also in elderly patients. It is feasible from a technical perspective, despite the fact that the brain is tighter at the time of early surgery, since the dissection of the aneurysm did not appear to be more difficult and the incidence of premature leak or rupture is the same compared to late surgery [12]. Since more than half of our patients were graded Fisher 4, i.e. with intracerebral hemorrhage, an early operation combined with removal of the space-occupying lesion is often necessary also from that point of view. The risk of rebleeding was reported to be 12% within 2 weeks after the initial hemorrhage [12] and that rate can be reduced markedly. None of our patients had a rebleeding after surgical clipping. Early surgery cannot prevent vasospasm, but the intensive care management, e.g. triple-H-therapy, is much easier and safer in patients with clipped aneurysms compared to those without, especially regarding the risk of rebleeding.

Since the outcome of conservatively managed elderly patients with ruptured cerebral aneurysms is very poor [5] we think that surgical treatment should not be refused only on the basis of advanced age. It has also been shown, that surgery on elderly patients with unruptured aneurysms can be done safely with low mortality and morbidity [9], therefore age alone should not exclude patients from surgical treatment. There is the chance of a good outcome after early surgery, especially in patients who are in good clinical conditions, in patients without excessive atherosclerotic changes in the angiography, and in those with aneurysms of the AcoA, also in this patient group. On the other hand, according to our results, surgery on patients HH 5 should be done only if clinical condition has improved after a period of stabilization.

References

1. Bailes JE, Spetzler RF, Hadley MN, Baldwin HZ (1990) Management morbidity and mortality of poor-grade aneurysm patients. J Neurosurg 72: 559–566
2. Broderick JP, Brott T, Tomsick T, Miller R, Huster G (1993) Intracerebral hemorrhage more than twice as common as subarachoid hemorrhage. J Neurosurg 78: 188–191
3. Chung RY, Carter BS, Norbash A, Budzik R, Putman C, Ogilvy CS (2000) Management outcomes for ruptured and unruptured aneurysms in the elderly. Neurosurgery 47: 827–833
4. Fisher CM, Kistler JP, Davis JM (1980) Relation of cerebral vasospasm to subarachnoid hemorrhage visualized by CT scanning. Neurosurgery 6: 1–9
5. Fridriksson SM, Hillman J, Saveland H, Brandt L (1995) Intracranial aneurysms surgery in the 8th and 9th decades of life: impact on population-based management outcome. Neurosurgery 37: 627–632
6. Hop JW, Rinkel GJE, Algra A, van Gijn J (1996) Case-fatality rates and functional outcome after subarachnoid hemorrhage. A systemic review. Stroke 28: 660–664
7. Hunt WE, Hess RM (1968) Surgical risk as related to time of intervention in the repair of intracranial aneurysms. J Neurosurg 28: 14–20
8. Inagawa T, Yamamoto M, Kamiya K, Ogasawara H (1988) Management of elderly patients with subarachnoid hemorrhage. J Neurosurg 69: 332–339
9. Inagawa T, Hada H, Katoh Y (1992) Unruptured intracranial aneurysms in elderly patients. Surg Neurol 38: 364–370
10. Inagawa T (1993) Management outcome in the elderly patient following subarachnoid hemorrhage. J Neurosurg 78: 554–561
11. Kassel NF, Torner JC, Haley C, Jane JA, Adams H, Kongable GL, and participants (1990) The international cooperative study on the timing of aneurysm surgery. Part 1: overall management results. J Neurosurg 73: 18–36
12. Kassel NF, Torner JC, Jane JA, Haley EC, Adams HP, and participants (1990) The international cooperative study on the timing of aneurysm surgery. Part 2: surgical results. J Neurosurg 73: 37–47
13. Lanzino G, Kassel NF, Germanson TP, Kongable GL, Truskowski LL, Torner J, Jane JA, the participants (1996) Age and outcome after aneurysmal subarachnoid hemorrhage: why do older patients fare worse? J Neurosurg 85: 410–418
14. Le Roux PD, Elliott JP, Newell DW, Grady MS, Winn HR (1996) Prediciting outcome in poor-grade patients with subarachnoid hemorrhage: a retrospective review of 159 aggressively managed cases. J Neurosurg 85: 39–49
15. Longstreth Jr WT, Koepsell TD, Yerby MS, van Belle G (1985) Risk factors for subarachnoid hemorrhage. Stroke 16: 377–386
16. Melamed E, Lavy S, Bentin S, Cooper G, Rinot Y (1980) Reduction in cerebral blood flow during normal aging in man. Stroke 11: 31–35
17. Sacco RL, Wolf PA, Bharucha NE ET AL (1984) Subarachnoid and intracerebral hemorrhage: natural history, prognosis, and precursive factors in the Framingham Study. Neurology 34: 847–854
18. Yamashita K, Kashiwagi S, Kato S, Takasago T, Ito H (1997) Cerebral aneurysms in the elderly in Yamaguchi, Japan. Analysis of the Yamaguchi data bank of cerebral aneurysms from 1985 to 1995. Stroke 28: 1926–1931

Correspondence: Prof. Dr. Ch. B. Lumenta, Department of Neurosurgery, Academic Hospital Munich-Bogenhausen, Technical University of Munich, Englschalkingerstr. 77, 81925 Munich, Germany.

Acta Neurochir (2002) [Suppl] 82: 65–69
© Springer-Verlag 2002

Clinical Outcome Following Ultra-Early Operation for Patients with Intracerebral Hematoma from Aneurysm Rupture – Focussing on the Massive Intra-Sylvian Type of Subarachnoid Hemorrhage

C.-C. Su[1], **K. Saito**[1], **A. Nakagawa**[1], **T. Endo**[1], **Y. Suzuki**[1], and **R. Shirane**[2]

[1] Department of Neurosurgery, Prefectural Shinjo Hospital, Yamagata, Japan
[2] Department of Neurosurgery, Tohoku University, Sendai, Japan

Summary

Of 250 patients admitted with aneurysmal subarachnoid hemorrhage (SAH) from 1994 to 2000, 16 had massive intra-sylvian hematomas. To predict the useful determinants of the clinical outcome for such patients we analyzed our last 16 cases. The study was performed in 2 parts. Part 1 covered the period from 1994 to 1996 and included 5 patients who underwent early surgery. Immediately before operation, Hunt & Kosnik grade (H&K) III was observed in 1, IV in 3 and V in 1 patient. Part 2, from 1997 to 2000, included 11 patients who underwent ultra-early surgery (within 3 hours after admission) with ventriculostomy and with 2 weeks' postoperative management in the ICU. Preoperatively, there were 2 patients with H&K III, 7 with IV, and 2 with V. The results in part 1 showed that 3 out of the 5 patients had poor outcome with symptomatic vasospasm. While in Part 2, seven returned to work, 2 had minimal and 1 had severe neurological deficits with symptomatic vasospasm, and 1 died. We therefore suggest that ultra-early surgery with ventriculostomy and postoperative management in the ICU is the most useful determinant to improve the clinical outcome in the treatment of SAH patients with massive intra-sylvian hematoma.

Keywords: SAH; intra-sylvian hematoma; and ultra-early operation.

Introduction

There is increasing evidence that early SAH operation improves the overall management results, particularly for SAH patients with significant hematoma [4, 6, 7]. However, even when performed as an early procedure, results remain poor in SAH patients with massive intra-sylvian hematoma [5, 8]. To find out which surgical techniques and postoperative management for such patients are predictors of the clinical outcome; we analyzed our last 16 cases. Of the 16 patients, 5 underwent early surgery (within 18 hours after admission) and 11 patients underwent ultra-early

surgery (within 3 hours after admission) with ventriculostomy and with 2 weeks' postoperative management in the ICU. In this study the clinical manifestations, the important role of ultra-early operation, and the essence of postoperative management in the ICU for such patients, are described, followed by a review of the literature and discussion of the different results between these 2 groups.

Materials and Methods

During the last 5 years (from November 1994 to December 2000), we experienced a series of 250 SAH patients. SAH with massive sylvian ICH was observed in 19 patients. Among the total 250 SAH patients, 228 were treated surgically. We excluded 3 cases complicated by massive intra-sylvian hematoma that showed no brain-stem reaction when admitted to our unit. Of the surgically treated 228 patients, SAH with massive intra-sylvian ICH was observed in 16 patients. The preoperative examination methods of the aneurysms were as follows: using DSA in 9, 3D Angio-CT in 4 and CT only in 3 patients.

Four males and 12 females with a mean age of 65.2 were operated on in our hospital (Table 1). The study was performed in 2 parts. Part 1 covered the period from November 1994 to December 1996 and included 5 patients who underwent early surgery (within 18 hours

Table 1. *Subjects and Methods in this Study*

Part 1 (Nov. 1994–Dec. 1996)
5 patients underwent acute surgery (within 18 hours after admission) without using ventriculostomy or performing management in the ICU.
Part 2 (Jan. 1997–Dec. 2000)
11 patients underwent ultra-early surgery (within 3 hours after admission) with ventriculostomy and 2 weeks postoperative managenent in the ICU.

Average age: 65.2 y.o; male : female = 4 : 12.

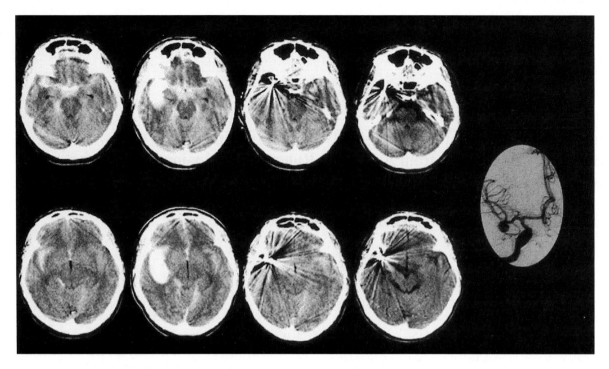

Fig. 1. CT scans in a 40-year-old male demonstrating re-rupture of a right middle cerebral aneurysm. The first row: On admission having H&K SAH grade II. The second row: Immediately after a CT scan showing rebleeding with massive intra-sylvian hematoma. The third row: CT scans after an ultra-early operation. The fourth row: He returned to work 2 months after admission

after admission) without using ventriculostomy or performing management in the ICU. Immediately before operation, Hunt & Kosnik grade (H&K) III was observed in 1, IV in 3 and V in 1 patient. Part 2, from January 1997 to December 2000, included 11 patients who underwent ultra-early surgery (within 3 hours) with ventriculostomy and with 2 weeks' postoperative management in the ICU. Preoperatively, there were 2 patients with H&K III, 7 with IV, and 2 with V. Postoperative hypertension did not occur and hypervolemia therapy was not performed in the 2 parts.

Results

The re-rupture rate of the aneurysms was 50%, that is, 8 out of the 16 patients had clinical evidence of re-rupture from aneurysms (Fig. 1). Of the re-ruptured cases (Table 2a), 2 were observed at home, 3 were in an ambulance car, 1 was in the emergency room, 1 was observed immediately after a CT scan, and 1 was when during transportation in the hospital. However, emergent DSA, tracheal intubation, and Foley catheter insertion were not the risk factor of aneurysmal re-rupture.

In summary of the medical complications during hospitalization (Table 2b), we found anemia in 3, electrolytes disturbance in 5, hepatic and/or renal dysfunction in 4, pathological arrhythmia in 2, congestive heart failure in 2, and pulmonary edema in 1, and pleural effusion in 3 patients.

Table 2a. *(Clinical Evidences of AN Re-Rupture)*

	8/16
At Home	2
In an ambulance	3
After arriving at the Hospital	
In the emergency room	1
Immediately after CT	1
During transportation in the hospital	1
During an emergent DSA	0
Tracheal intubation and Foley catheter insertion	0

Table 2b. *(Medical Complications During Hospitalization)*

Anemia	3	Pneumonia	2
Electrolyte disturbance	5	Congestive heart failure	2
Hepatic and/or renal dysfunct.	4	Pulmonary edema	1
Pathological arrhythmia	2	Pleural effusion	3

Functional outcomes 3 months after the onset of SAH were as follows; Part 1: Three of the 5 patients had poor outcome with symptomatic vasospasm; two died, and one had severe neurological deficits. Out of the remaining 2 patients, one had excellent outcome and one had good outcome. Part 2: One patient died. Out of the remaining 10 patients, 7 returned to work (Fig. 2), 2 had minimal neurological deficits (Fig. 3),

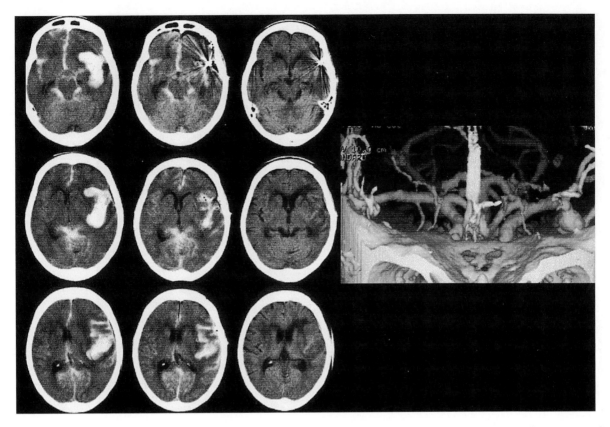

Fig. 2. CT and 3D Angio-CT scans in a 71-year-old female demonstrating SAH with massive intra-sylvian hematoma due to rupture of a left middle cerebral aneurysm. The first row: On admission having H&K SAH grade IV. The second row: Ultra-early surgery was performed immediately after a 3D Angio-CT scan. The third row: She left hospital with good recovery 7 weeks after admission

and 1 was in bed-ridden state due to symptomatic vasospasm.

Discussion

Patients with massive ICH secondary to aneurysm bleeding have a poor prognosis if not treated early [1, 4, 5, 6]. At present, emergent CT with 3D Angio-CT is increasingly used as the first diagnostic tool in vascular catastrophes due to the innovation of helical CT scan, and an increasing tendency towards early or emergent treatment of aneurysmal hematoma is thus reported. According to the distribution of SAH hematomas, ruptured middle cerebral artery (MCA) aneurysms can be divided into two patterns: the temporal intra-parenchymal and the intra-sylvian hematomas [7, 8]. In the literature, it is suggested that temporal intra-parenchymal hematoma from rupture of an MCA aneurysm has the potential to achieve a good prognosis if treated emergently, particularly in younger patients. However, even when performed as an early procedure, results remain poor in SAH patients with massive intra-sylvian hematoma [5, 7, 8]. Yoshimoto et al. [8] accurately assessed a series of 24 SAH patients suffering from massive intra-sylvian ICH and found 54% and 50% of patients complicated by subsequent brain edema and symptomatic vasospasm, respectively. They concluded that an accurate assessment of the bleeding patterns in patients with ruptured MCA aneurysms would be necessary in helping neuro-surgeons predict the clinical course and the most appropriate treatment. Batjer et al. [1] and Tapaninaho et al. [7] even stated the important role to perform emergent aneurysm surgeries without cerebral angiography for the treatment of such critical patients, although the functional outcomes remained poor.

To achieve good overall management results for such patients, many studies focussing on the timing of aneurysm surgery have been documented in the literature. However, little attention has been paid to the other predictors that can also influence the overall outcome, such as surgical techniques, perioperative medical complications, and postoperative management in the ICU. In this study, we analyzed our last 16

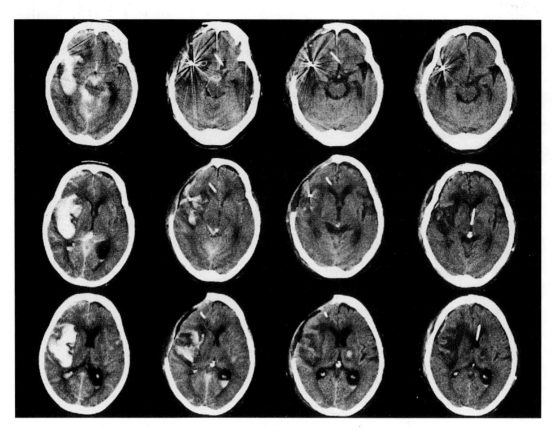

Fig. 3. This case shows a 68-year-old female having H&G SAH grade V when admitted. The first row: CT scans on admission showing SAH with massive intra-sylvian hematoma. The second row: Immediately after an ultra-early operation demonstrating evacuation of the hematoma with ventriculostomy and with outer decompression. The third row: Three weeks after operation, a small left thalamic hemorrhage occurred. The fourth row: Three weeks after a VP shunt and 2 months later after a cranioplasty, she recovered well with a very mild right hemiparesis

cases to assess the predictors for improving clinical outcome. Of the 16 patients, group 1 included 5 patients who underwent early surgery (within 18 hours after admission) and group 2 included 11 patients undergoing ultra-early surgery (within 3 hours after admission) with ventriculostomy and with 2 weeks' postoperative management in the ICU. The preoperative H&K grading in part 1 and part 2 was observed to be of the same distribution. However, the functional outcomes, 3 months after onset of SAH, were as follows; Part 1: Three of the 5 patients had poor outcome with symptomatic vasospasm; two died, and one had severe neurological deficits. From the remaining 2 patients, one had excellent outcome and one had good outcome. Part 2: One patient died. Out of the remaining 10 patients, 7 returned to work, 2 had minimal neurological deficits, and 1 was in bed-ridden state due to symptomatic vasospasm. The results indicate that ultra-early surgery with ventriculostomy is essential and can obtain a good prognosis in most patients in part 2

(GOS 1: 7/11, GOS 2: 2/11). Moreover, preoperative tracheal intubation due to respiratory failure was performed in 8 patients (50%) of each group. As medical complications during hospitalization were observed: anemia in 3, electrolytes disturbance in 5, hepatic and/ or renal dysfunction in 4, pathological arrhythmia in 2, congestive heart failure in 2, and pulmonary edema in 1, and pleural effusion in 3 patients. Because of the strict postoperative management in the ICU, none of the patients had permanent medical complications in the follow-up periods. This also indicates that a strict postoperative management in the ICU for the treatment of SAH patients with massive intra-sylvian hematoma is important.

Aneurysmal re-rupture was found in 8 out of the 16 patients (50%) in this study. Of the re-ruptured cases, 2 were observed at home, 3 were in an ambulance car, 1 was in the emergency room, 1 was observed immediately after a CT scan, and 1 was during transportation in the hospital. However, emergent DSA, tracheal intubation, and Foley catheter insertion were not the risk factor for aneurysmal re-rupture. The high rate of aneurysmal re-rupture before arriving at hospital indicates that an initial management such as sedation and using anti-hypertensive agents for suspicious SAH patients is essential. It is also helpful to know the clinical course and the most appropriate management for SAH patients before and immediately after arriving at hospital.

According to our experience ultra-early surgery with ventriculostomy and postoperative management in the ICU is the most important to improve the clinical outcome in the treatment of SAH patients with massive intra-sylvian hematoma.

Conclusion

It is difficult to perform ultra-early surgery in most neurosurgical units, and the postoperative management of choice for these patients is also difficult to assess. However, we suggest that ultra-early surgery with ventriculostomy and postoperative management in the ICU may be essential to improve the clinical outcome in the treatment of SAH patients with significant sylvian ICH.

References

1. Batjer HH, Samson DS (1991) Emergent aneurysm surgery without cerebral angiography for the comatose patient. Neurosurgery 28(2): 283–287
2. Hosoda K, Fujita S, Kawaguchi T, Shose Y, Hamano S, Iwakura M (1999) Effect of clot removal and surgical manipulation on regional cerebral blood flow and delayed vasospasm in early aneurysm surgery for subarachnoid hemorrhage. Surg Neurol 51(1): 81–88
3. Inagawa T, Yamamoto M, Kamiya K (1990) Effect of clot removal on cerebral vasospasm. J Neurosurg 72(2): 224–230
4. Ljunggren B, Saveland H, Brandt L, Zygmunt S (1985) Early operation and overall outcome in aneurysmal subarachnoid hemorrhage. J Neurosurg 62(4): 547–551
5. Nowak G, Schwachenwald D, Schwachenwald R, Kehler U, Muller H, Arnold H (1998) Intracerebral hematomas caused by aneurysm rupture. Experience with 67 cases. Neurosurg Rev 21(1): 5–9
6. Takahashi S, Sonobe M, Nagamine Y (1981) Early operations for ruptured intracranial aneurysms – comparative study with computed tomography. No Shinkei Geka 9(2): 151–156
7. Tapaninaho A, Hernesniemi J, Vapalahti M (1988) Emergency treatment of cerebral aneurysms with large haematomas. Acta Neurochir (Wien) 91(1–2): 21–24
8. Yoshimoto Y, Wakai S, Satoh A, Hirose Y (1999) Intaparenchymal and intrasylvian haematomas secondary to ruptured middle cerebral artery aneurysms: prognostic factors and therapeutic considerations. Br J Neurosurg 13(1): 18–24

Correspondence: Ching-Chan Su, M.D., Department of Neurosurgery, Prefectural Shinjo Hospital, Wakabamachi 12-55, Shinjo City, Yamagata Prefecture, 996-0025 Japan.

Acta Neurochir (2002) [Suppl] 82: 71–81
© Springer-Verlag 2002

Presentation and Management of Patients with Initial Negative 4-Vessel Cerebral Angiography in Subarachnoid Hemorrhage

N. Khan[1], **B. Schuknecht**[2], and **Y. Yonekawa**[1]

[1] Department of Neurosurgery, University Hospital Zurich, Zurich, Switzerland
[2] Department of Neuroradiology, University Hospital Zurich, Zurich, Switzerland

Summary

The importance of repeat-angiography in patients with acute sub-arachnoid hemorrhage (SAH) and initial negative angiography has been reviewed in the light of our patient population (19 patients with initial negative angiography/168 patients with SAH). The type of SAH i.e., nontraumatic perimesencephalic SAH versus focal or generalized non perimesencephalic SAH, as well as the amount and distribution of blood on the initial CT examination are important factors in decision making. 3D-Angio-CT, in 3/5 patients, and MR-angiography (MRA) in 1/5 patients were complementary non-invasive methods to diagnose aneurysms on repeated examinations. Repeat-cerebral angiography confirmed the source of hemorrhage in 3 patients.

Keywords: Four vessel cerebral angiography; 3D-Angio-CT; MR-angiography; Subarachnoid hemorrhage; intracranial aneurysms.

Introduction

Subarachnoid hemorrhage (SAH) results from rupture of cerebral aneurysms in 80% of the cases. Four-vessel cerebral angiography remains the gold standard in identifying cerebral aneurysms in the light of acute subarachnoid hemorrhage. The incidence of initial negative angiography in patients with SAH ranges between 15%–20% and repeat angiographies have been able to diagnose aneurysms in 0%–20% of the cases [4, 9, 13, 17]. The question that still remains open to us is therefore the definition of a protocol of investigation, treatment and follow-up to execute in cases of initial negative angiographies in patients with acute non-perimesencephalic SAH. We therefore examined the incidence of initial negative angiography in our group of patients with SAH and reviewed the efficacy of repeat angiography in detection and diagnosis of ruptured/unruptured aneurysms in these cases. The clinical pre-sentation and management of these patients is presented.

Materials and Methods

During the period of July 1998–November 2000, 168 patients with acute SAH were treated in our neurosurgical department. The diagnosis of acute SAH was made on CT examination in all but one case. In this case the diagnosis was made on the basis of a positive hemorrhagic lumbar puncture. To define the exact source of bleeding initial four-vessel cerebral angiography was performed in all patients.

We examined the clinical presentation in terms of the Hunt and Hess and WFNS grading, type of SAH i.e. non-traumatic acute SAH versus perimesencephalic SAH and intensity of SAH on CT images in terms of the Fisher grading. Repeat cerebral angiography was performed in 10 patients. Initial 3D-Angio-CT and MR-angiography were performed additionally, complementary to the cerebral angiography, in 5 cases.

Results

Four-vessel cerebral angiography was negative in 19/168 of the patients presenting with SAH on CT. Six of these 19 patients presented with a perimesencephalic type of SAH. The Fisher grading at initial presentation was as follows: Grade I: n = 1, Grade II: n = 4, Grade III: n = 6, Grade IV: n = 2.

Repeat angiography was performed in 9 of the 168 patients with non-perimesencephalic SAH with initial negative findings. The Fisher grading in these patients was as follows: Grade II: n = 3, Grade III: n = 5, Grade IV: n = 1. Only in one patient with a peri-mesencephalic SAH with negative initial angiography, a repeat-angiography was performed within one week. One patient with a negative CT and positive hemorrhagic lumbar puncture underwent a repeat angiography 4 months after the initial negative angiography due to a suspicious finding on MRA.

Examining the initial clinical and neuroradiological presentation of our patient group we were able to divide them into four subgroups:

Group 1: patients with clear SAH on CT, negative initial angiography, positive repeat angiography, Group 2: perimesencephalic SAH with negative angiography, Group 3: SAH of Fisher grade II or more with negative initial and negative repeated angiography and Group 4: SAH of Fisher grade II or more with suspicion of aneurysm on initial angiography and negative repeat angiography.

Group 1: Patients with Clear SAH on CT, Negative Initial Angiography, Positive Repeat Angiography

Three patients showed aneurysms on second angiography.

Case 1: WE 40 Y F

Forty year old female patient presented with SAH Day 0, Hunt Hess I, Fisher III, WFNS III.

Initial 4-vessel cerebral angiography and a 3D-Angio-CT were negative. After 40 minutes of initial presentation, the patient deteriorated clinically showing a Hunt Hess grade of V, Fisher III and WFNS V. A repeat-angiography and 3D-Angio-CT demonstrated an A1-aneurysm. Intraoperatively a broad-based dissection A1 aneurysm, partly thrombosed, was observed and clipped. Inspite of all possible therapeutic measures, the patient maintained a constant increased intracranial pressure and died a week later.

Case 2: SH 68 Y F

Sixty-eight year old female patient presented with SAH Day 1, Hunt Hess III, Fisher II, WFNS III. Four-vessel cerebral angiography was negative for aneurysms. A suspicious widening of the MCA and Pcomm. on the left side was noticed which advocated exploration. Intraoperatively the exploration of the ICA, MCA and P comm did not reveal any aneurysm. Postoperatively the patient recovered clinically but required a ventriculo-peritoneal shunt due to post-SAH hydrocephalus. On day 17 the patient clinically deteriorated to a Hunt Hess score of V, Fisher IV and WFNS V. Repeat CT examination showed a repeat

SAH with intraventricular hemorrhage. An external ventricle drainage was performed and the angiography repeated. The repeat-angiography revealed a P comm. aneurysm. Intraoperatively a PCA aneurysm (P1–P2) with a relatively small neck was found and clipped. The patient did not recover clinically and died 2 weeks later of a multi-organ failure.

Case 3: HG 47 Y M

Forty-seven year old male patient presented with an episode of acute headache with spontaneous relief followed by a similar episode 7 days later which persisted from then on. The patient presented himself to the ER where a normal neurological status was found. CT scan of the head was also normal. A lumbar puncture performed on the same day was hemorrhagic. MRA performed on the ninth day and a 3D-Angio-CT performed on the 10th day revealed a suspicious finding at the location of the P. comm. Angiography performed on the 10th day did not confirm any aneurysmal finding. A follow-up repeat angiography performed 4 months after the initial angiography was positive for a recanalised, irregularly formed P. comm aneurysm of about 1 cm in size. The aneurysm was clipped and the patient showed an uneventful postoperative recovery and follow-up.

Group 2: Patients with Perimesencephalic SAH with Negative Angiography

Six of 19 patients presented with a perimesencephalic type of SAH. All but one patient presented with a Hunt Hess grade of II and WFNS grade of I.

This patient presented with SAH with intraventricular hemorrhage due to which initially an external ventricle drainage and later a ventriculoperitoneal shunt was performed. All patients had negative angiography, repeat MRA performed in 2 patients within a period of one week was negative. All patients showed favorable outcome.

Group 3: Patients with SAH of Fisher Grade II or More with Negative Initial and Negative Repeated Angiography

Case 1: FP 64 Y M

Sixty-four year old male patient presented with SAH, Day 0, Hunt Hess IV, Fisher III, WFNS V. CT showed additional hydrocephalus. Initial 4-vessel an-

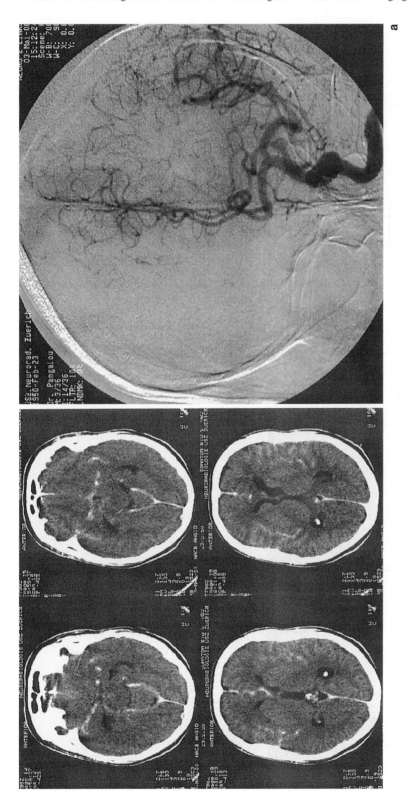

Fig. 1. (a) CT scan of patient WE 40Y F showing a diffuse SAH: Fisher grade III, initial 4-vessel cerebral angiography (left carotid injection) was negative for any aneurysm. (b) CT scan 40 minutes later showing a Fisher grade III (rebleeding), repeat-angiography showing A1-aneurysm

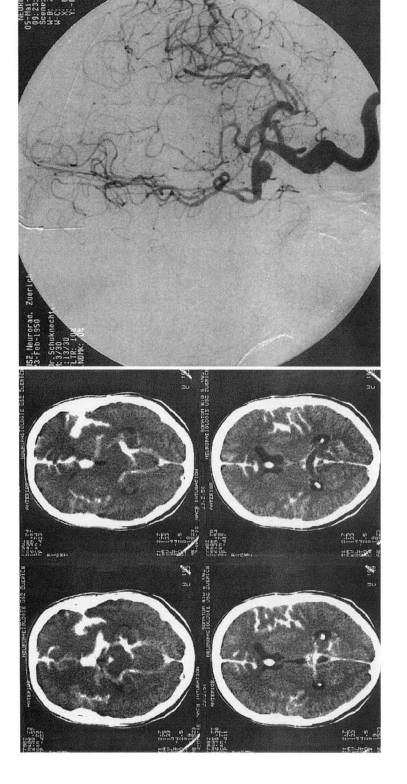

Fig. 1. (continued)

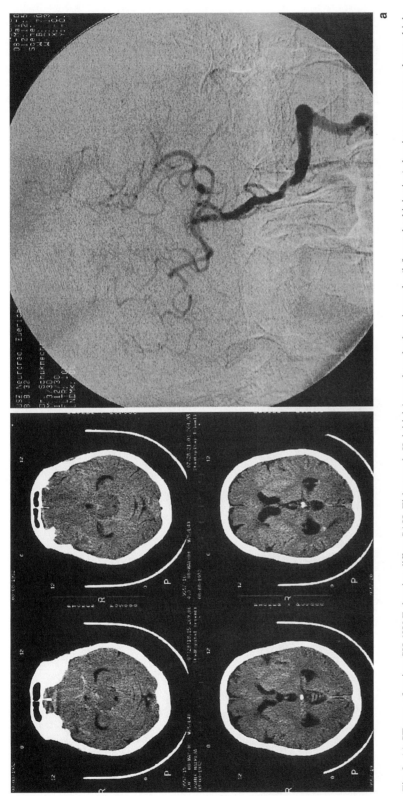

Fig. 2. (a) CT scan of patient SH 68Y F showing diffuse SAH: Fisher grade II, initial 4-vessel cerebral angiography (left vertebral injection) showing no aneurysm but multiple stenotic lesions and irregularities. (b) On Day 17, CT scan with Fisher grade IV and repeat-angiography showing PCA aneurysm

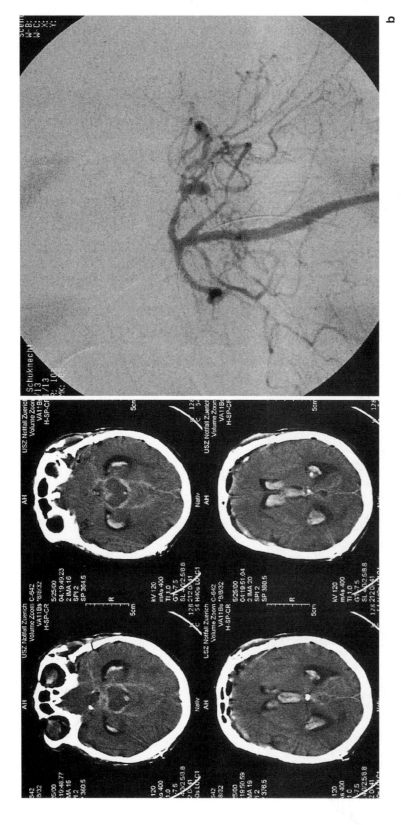

Fig. 2. (continued)

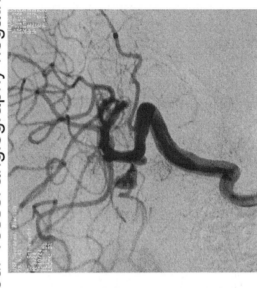

Four-vessel angiography negative

Repeat angiography positive

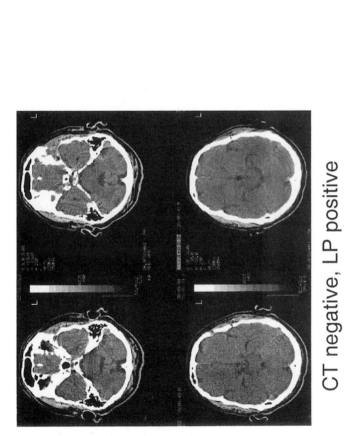

CT negative, LP positive

MRA suspicion of Pcomm. aneurysm

Fig. 3. Patient HG 47Y M: initial CT scan was normal, MRA showed suspicion of P Comm. aneurysm, initial 4-vessel angiography was negative, repeat angiography 4 months later confirmed a P Comm. aneurysm

giography and 3D-Angio-CT were negative. An external ventricle drainage was performed and could be removed within a few days. A repeat angiography performed 10 days after the SAH remained negative for any aneurysms. Follow-up was uneventful.

Case 2: NP

A 59 year old male patient presented with SAH Hunt Hess II, Fisher IV, WFNS I. Initial angiography was negative for the source of bleeding. Two days after initial presentation the patient deteriorated clinically due to a decompensated hydrocephalus for which a ventriculo-peritoneal shunt was placed. The patient recovered immediately and follow-up was unremarkable. A repeat angiography performed a week later was also negative for any aneurysms.

Group 4: Patients with SAH of Fisher Grade II or More with Suspicion of Aneurysm on Initial Angiography and Negative Repeat Angiography

Case 1: EV 55 Y M

A fifty-five year old male patient presented with SAH, Day 0, Hunt Hess III, Fisher IV, WFNS IV. CT showed a right frontal intracerebral hematoma additionally. Initial 4-vessel cerebral angiography and 3D-Angio-CT suggested the possibility of a right MCA aneurysm. Operative exploration and hematoma evacuation could not confirm the presence of an MCA aneurysm. A wall weakness at the MCA bifurcation was noticed and this was strengthened with muscle coating. A repeat angiography performed 11 days postoperatively was still negative. Postoperatively the patient did well with an uneventful recovery and follow-up.

Discussion

The incidence of a negative angiogram in acute SAH ranges from 15% to 20% [4, 9, 13, 17]. In our patient group an incidence of 10% was seen. Some authors report a higher incidence of up to 31% with a false negative rate of 5% [8]. The exact percentage of false negative angiograms is difficult to assess in general since the number of repeat angiographies performed are different from patient population to patient population. In our patient group a repeated angiography was positive in 33% (3/9) of patients with non-perimesencephalic SAH. On the other hand there are

some authors who do not advocate repeat angiographies in SAH if the angiographies performed are technically good, carefully evaluated and there is no evidence of vasospasm [7, 10]. This reiterates the need of a protocol or algorithm in patient management in acute SAH with initial negative angiography failing to demonstrate the source of hemorrhage.

The importance of Fisher grading i.e. amount and distribution of blood on initial CT plays a crucial role in further management of these cases. Also the type of SAH i.e, nontraumatic acute SAH versus perimesencephalic type of SAH is also a key factor in management. PMH accounts for 21–68% of cases of angiography negative SAH [16] and in only 5% of cases posterior circulation aneurysms, mainly vertebrobasilar, are the cause of hemorrhage [18]. These cases have a good prognosis and no risk of rebleeding and a lesser risk of vasospasm compared to patients with SAH of unknown etiology [14, 16, 18]. A repeat angiography is advocated if the amount of blood on initial CT is large enough for a Fisher grade II or the initial angiography demonstrates a suspicious finding. Most of the PMH do not warrant a repeat angiography [14, 16]. MRA [1, 5, 11, 15] and 3D-Angio-CT [2, 3, 14, 19] are non-invasive investigations complementary to the cerebral angiography, specifying the indication of repeat angiography and allowing a better view of aneurysm morphology and their relation to the skull base.

A Fisher grading of II or more, especially with the presence of focal hemorrhage, considerable amount of blood in the interhemispheric fissure should increase the suspicion of an aneurysm in this location and warrant for repeat angiographies [4]. The increased number of missed anterior circulation aneurysms has also been mentioned in the literature [4, 12].

Keeping these patient subgroups in acute SAH with initial negative angiographies in mind we have outlined a protocol according to the type of SAH and Fisher grading in Fig. 5.

The cause of initial negative angiography in aneurysmal SAH is thought to be frequently due to acute thrombus formation with presence of an intra-aneurysmal clot as was the case in our 3 patients in group 1 [4]. Presence of vasospasm during the angiography can also result in missing an aneurysmal finding. SAH caused by microaneurysms [17] which represent saccular aneurysms with a small aneurysmal sac may also often be missed on initial angiography. These aneurysms have a tendency to enlarge over days, as

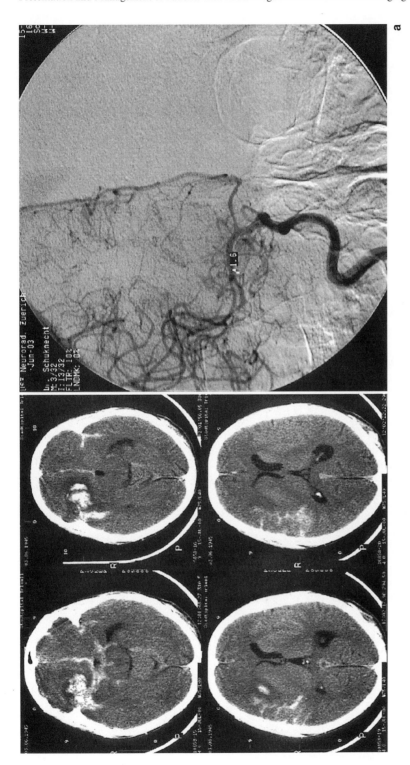

Fig. 4. (a) CT scan of patient EV 55Y M showing SAH with left sylvian preponderance as well as a right frontal intracerebral hematoma, suspicion of MCA aneurysm on initial angiography. (b) Repeat angiographies were negative

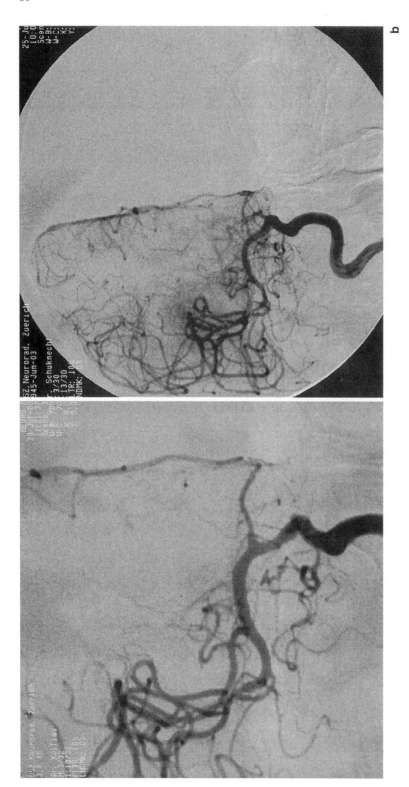

Fig. 4. (continued)

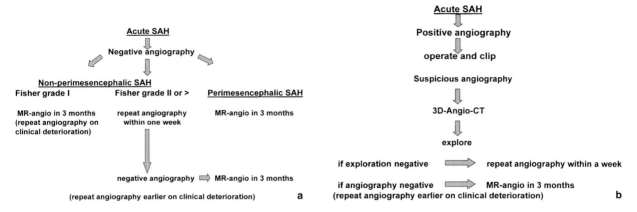

Fig. 5. (a, b) Protocol of management in acute SAH with initial negative angiography (a) and initial positive angiography (b)

was seen in one of our patients (HG 47Y M), and are usually detected incidentally but present with a significant risk of rebleeding.

References

1. Adams WM, Laitt RD, Jackson A (2000) The role of MR angiography in the pretreatment assessment of intracranial aneurysms: A comparative study. AJNR 21: 168–1628
2. Alberico RA, Patel M, Casey S, Jacob B, Maguire W, Decker R (1996) Evaluation of the circle of Willis with three-dimensional CT angiography in patients with suspected intracranial aneurysms. AJNR 17(5): 1002–1003
3. Anderson GB, Findlay JM, Steinke DE, Ashforth R (1997) Experience with computed tomographic angiography for the detection of intracranial aneurysms in the setting of acute subarachnoid hemorrhage. Neurosurgery 41(3): 522–528
4. Bradac GB, Bergui M, Ferrio MF, Fontanella M, Stura G (1997) False-negative angiograms in subarachnoid haemorrhage due to intracranial aneurysms. Neuroradiology 39: 772–776
5. Curnes JT, Shogry ME, Clark DC, Elsner HJ (1993) MR angiographic demonstration of an intracranial aneurysm not seen on conventional angiography. AJNR 14(4): 971–973
6. Di Lorenzo N, Guidetti G (1988) Anterior communicating aneurysm missed at angiography: report of two cases treated surgically. Neurosurgery 23(4): 494–499
7. du Mesnil de Rochemont R, Heindel W, Wesselmann C, Kruger K, Lanfermann H, Ernestus RI, Neveling M, Lackner K (1997) Nontraumatic subarachnoid hemorrhage: value of repeat angiography. Radiology 202(3): 798–800
8. Duong H, Melancon D, Tampieri D, Ethier R (1995) The negative angiogram in subarachnoid haemorrhage. Neuroradiology 38(1): 15–19
9. Farres MT, Ferraz-Leite H, Schindler E, Muhlbauer M (1992) Spontaneous subarachnoid hemorrhage with negative angiography findings. J Comput Assist Tomography 16(4): 534–537
10. Gilbert JW, Lee C, Young B (1990) Repeat cerebral pan- angiography in subarachnoid hemorrhage of unknown etiology. Surg Neurol 33(1): 19–21
11. Gouliamos A, Gotsis E, Vlahos L, Samara C, Kapsalaki E, Rologist Z, Papavasiliou C (1992) Magnetic resonance angiography compared to intra-arterial subtraction angiography in patients with subarachnoid hemorrhage. Neuroradiology 35(1): 46–49
12. Iwanaga H, Wakai S, Ochiai C, Narita J, Inoh S, Nagai M (1990) Ruptured cerebral aneurysms missed by initial angiographic study. Neurosurgery 27(1): 45–51
13. Kaim A, Proske M, Kirsch E, von Weymarn A, Radu EW (1996) Value of repeat-angiography in cases of unexplained subarachnoid hemorrhage. Acta Neurol Scand 93(5): 336–373
14. Ruigrok YM, Rinkel GJE, Buskens E, Velthuis BK, van Gijn J (2000) Perimesencephalic hemorrhage and CT angiography: A decision analysis. Stroke 31(12): 2976–2983
15. Schuierer G, Huk WJ, Laub G (1992) Magnetic resonance angiography of the intracranial aneurysms: comparison with intra-arterial digital subtraction angiography. Neuroradiology 35(1): 50–54
16. Schwarz TH, Solomon RA (1996) Perimesencephalic non-aneurysmal subarachnoid hemorrhage; Review of literature. Neurosurgery 39: 433–440
17. Tatter SB, Crowell RM, Ogilvy CS (1995) Aneurysmal and microaneurysmal "angiogram-negative" subarachnoid hemorrhage. Neurosurgery 37: 48–55
18. Velthuis BK, Rinkel GJE, Ramos LMP, Witkamp TD, van Leeuwen MS (1999) Perimesencephalic hemorrhage: Exclusion of vertebrobasilar aneurysms with CT angiography. Stroke 30: 1103–1109
19. Zouaoui A, Sahel M, Marro B, Clemenceau S, Dargent N, Bitar A, Faillot T, Capelle L, Marsault C (1997) Three-dimensional computed tomographic angiography in detection of cerebral aneurysms in acute subarachnoid hemorrhage. Neurosurgery 41(1): 125–130

Correspondence: Nadia Khan M.D., Department of Neurosurgery, University Hospital Zurich, Frauenklinikstrasse 10, 8091 Zurich, Switzerland.

Acta Neurochir (2002) [Suppl] 82: 83–85

Neurological and Neuropsychological Outcome after SAH

M. Bjeljac[1], **E. Keller**[1], **M. Regard**[2], and **Y. Yonekawa**[1]

[1] Department of Neurosurgery, University Hospital Zurich, Zurich, Switzerland
[2] Neuropsychology Unit, Department of Neurology, University Hospital Zurich, Zurich, Switzerland

Summary

The fact that neurological status and physical integrity alone do not sufficiently assess the overall state of patients after aneurysmal subarachnoid hemorrhage (SAH) gives rise to the necessity for complementary neuropsychological investigation. Neuropsychological work-up should also cover an emotional state, psychosocial adjustment and competence in everyday life of the patients. In our prospective study we investigated 82 patients three months and one year after SAH and early clipping of the aneurysm. For the evaluation of postoperative neurological functions the Glasgow Outcome Scale (GOS) was used. For the neuropsychological assessment we used standardized measures of verbal and figural learning and memory, verbal and figural fluency, speed of information processing, visuospacial abilities and affective function. One year after SAH 95.6% of patients with Hunt&Hess Grade 1 and 2 on admission showed good neurological results (GOS 4 and 5). However, only 30.1% (18 of 63 patients with a favourable neurological outcome – GOS 4 and 5) did not show any neuropsychological deficit. Localization of the ruptured aneurysm significantly correlated with cognitive measures. The best cognitive outcome was shown in patients with aneurysms on the anterior communicating artery (ACoA) followed by posterior communicating artery (PCoA) and those located on the internal carotid artery (ICA) on the right side.

Keywords: Subarachnoid hemorrhage; aneurysm rupture; outcome; cognitive deficits.

Introduction

The modern microsurgical techniques, the concept of early surgery and specialized intensive care units with pre- and postoperative management including standardized treatment regimen for cerebral vasospasm (consisting of hypertensive hypervolemic hemodilution, so called "Triple-H therapy", angioplasty and/or intraarterial superselective papaverine instillation and mild hypothermia as well as barbiturate coma if conventional treatment modalities were unsuccessful) have reduced mortality and morbidity of the patients with SAH. For the evaluation of the functional outcome after aneurysmal SAH, the GOS is most frequently used. As the GOS is restricted only to the dimensions of neurological integrity and physical independence it must be doubted that it is really a suitable instrument for measuring the overall state of patients functioning. In many studies it has been shown that patients after rupture and surgical therapy of an intracranial aneurysm exhibit substantial cognitive deficits and emotional problems although their neurological outcome had been rated as good [2, 3, 9, 11, 12]. For this reason complementary neuropsychological investigation and the health-related quality of life (QOL) must be integrated in the rating of postoperative outcome [5].

Material and Methods

From July 1998 to February 2000, 86 patients underwent surgery for a ruptured intracranial aneurysm in the Department of Neurosurgery, University Hospital Zurich. The patients had sustained aneurysmal SAH, documented by the results of cranial CT scanning (in all patients) and by lumbar puncture (in several patients). Four-vessel angiography excluded the presence of any vascular malformation other than an aneurysm, and no other cause of bleeding was identifiable. The severity of SAH was classified according to the Fisher CT grading system, and neurological condition on admission to the neurosurgical unit was rated according to the grading scale of Hunt and Hess (H&H) and the Word Federation of Neurological Surgeons (WFNS) scale. In all patients early clipping of the aneursym within 3 days was performed. In addition to the ruptured aneurysm, four-vessel angiography revealed another unruptured aneurysm in 12 patients (13.9%) and two unruptured aneurysms in 5 patients (5.8%). In 3 patients (3.5%) a giant aneurysm was found. These additional aneurysms were successfully clipped during the operation for the ruptured aneurysm. Postoperatively, all patients were treated according to a standardized protocol with nimodipine for three weeks and daily transcranial Doppler sonography. If mean transcranial Doppler blood flow velocities increased >100 cm/s, Triple-H therapy (hypertensive hypervolemic hemodilution) was initiated [7]. If the patients developed symptomatic CVS with signs of delayed ischemic neurologic deficit despite of maximal

Table 1. *Neuropsychological Test Procedures for Postoperative Evaluation*

Cognitive function	Neuropsychological test
Aphasia screening	Tocken-Test
Concentration	d2-Test
Interference	Stroop-Test
Verbal fluency	Verb generation
Non-verbal fluency	5 point-Test
Verbal learning and memory	10 words by Rey
Figural learning and memory	Rey-Osterrieth figure
Visuospatial ability	Modified Hooper-Test

Triple-H therapy, they were treated with angioplasty and/or selective papaverine infusion into the vasospastic vessels [6]. Patients with CVS resistant to two sessions of papaverine infusion were treated with barbiturate coma and/or mild hypothermia.

Of 86 patients 3 (3.5%) died during the acute phase of their illness.

Of the remaining 83 patients one patient had moved without leaving a forwarding address. Finally 82 patients available for the study underwent extensive neurological and neuropsychological examination at 3 and 12 months after aneurysm clipping. For the evaluation of postoperative neurological functions the Glasgow Outcome Scale (GOS) was used. The neuropsychological assessment consisted of standardized measures of verbal and figural learning and memory, verbal and non-verbal fluency, speed of information processing and visuospatial abilities (Table 1). For the evaluation of the quality of life and affective function we used a clinical interview.

Results

Compared to the status on admission all patients improved sensory-motor as well as executive functions 3 and 12 months postoperatively. Three months after

operation 92% of patients showed neurological improvements and 74% of patients showed cognitive improvements in at least one area of cognition. Twelve months after operation all patients showed significant improvements in neurological and neuropsychological status. Patients initially scored at grade 1 and 2 H&H scale were found to have a favorable neurological and neuropsychological outcome, thus confirming previous studies. Table 2 gives an overview of the correlation between H&H grade on admission and GOS three and twelve months after SAH.

However, one year after SAH only 30.1% (19 of 63 patients with a favourable neurological outcome – GOS 4 and 5) did not exhibit any neuropsychological deficit. Sixteen (25.4%) of patients presented with one and 17 (26.9%) of patients with two cognitive deficits. In 11 (17.5%) of patients three and more cognitive functions impaired. The best cognitive outcome was shown in patients with aneurysms on the anterior communicating artery (ACoA) followed by those located on posterior communicating artery (PCoA) and internal carotid artery on the right side. Table 3 gives an overview of the neuropsychological functions of patients with a good postoperative outcome (GOS 4 and 5) 12 months after SAH.

Discussion

In accordance with previous papers our study demonstrated impairments of short-term memory, atten-

Table 2. *H&H Grade vs. GOS in 82 Consecutively Treated Patients 3 and 12 Months after SAH*

	no. of patients (%)	Good recovery GOS 5		Moderate disability GOS 4		Severe disability GOS 2 + 3	
		3 Mt.	12 Mt.	3 Mt.	12 Mt.	3 Mt.	12 Mt.
All patients	82 (100%)	32 (39.0%)	40 (48.8%)	23 (28.0%)	23 (28.0%)	27 (32.9%)	19 (23.2%)
H&H 1 + 2	46 (56.1%)	30 (65.2%)	35 (76.1%)	12 (26.1%)	9 (19.5%)	4 (8.7%)	2 (4.3%)
H&H 3	12 (14.6%)	2 (16.7%)	3 (25.0%)	3 (25.0%)	5 (41.7%)	7 (58.3%)	4 (33.3%)
H&H 4	14 (17.1%)	0	1 (7.1%)	5 (35.7%)	6 (42.9%)	9 (64.3%)	7 (50.0%)
H&H 5	10 (12.2%)	0	1 (10.0%)	3 (30.0%)	4 (40.0%)	7 (70.0%)	5 (50.0%)

Table 3. *Cognitive Deficits of Patients with a Good Postoperative Outcome (GOS 4 and 5) 12 Months after SAH*

Cognitive deficits	ACoA no. (%) total 29	PCoA no. (%) total 8	MCA right no. (%) total 8	MCA left no. (%) total 6	ICA right no. (%) total 4	ICA left no. (%) total 3	other location no. (%) total 5
No deficits	11 (37.9%)	3 (37.5%)	1 (12.5%)	1 (16.7%)	1 (25.0%)	0	2 (40.0%)
1 deficit	8 (27.6%)	2 (25.0%)	2 (25.0%)	1 (16.7%)	2 (50.0%)	0	1 (20.0%)
2 deficits	7 (24.1%)	2 (25.0%)	2 (25.0%)	2 (33.3%)	1 (25.0%)	2 (66.7%)	1 (20.0%)
3 and more deficits	3 (10.3%)	1 (12.5%)	3 (37.5%)	2 (33.3%)	0	1 (33.3%)	1 (20.0%)

tion, concentration, cognitive speed and flexibility as the most frequent long-term sequelae of SAH [1, 2, 12]. Older patients (>60 years) were at follow-up significantly more disturbed in concentration, short-term memory and information processing capacity as compared to patients aged less than 60 years [4, 8]. Localization of the ruptured aneurysm significantly correlated with cognitive measures [2, 12, 13]. We found the best cognitive outcomes in patients with ACoA aneurysms. However, many previous reports showed more severe neuropsychological impairments – especially in memory functions – in patients with ACoA aneurysms compared to patients with ruptured aneurysms at other locations [14, 15]. Our findings of an overall favourable and a superior outcome may be related to microsurgical techniques as well as to the standardized treatment strategies of CVS on the neurocritical care unit. Our follow-up study up to one year after SAH showed marked sensory-motor improvements whereas cognitive functions only partially recovered. Therefore, Glasgow Outcome Score alone is insufficient for follow-up studies in patients after SAH.

References

1. Barbarotto R, De Santis A, Basso A, Spagnoli D, Capitani E (1989) Neuropsychological follow-up of patients operated for aneurysms of the middle cerebral artery and posterior communicating artery. Cortex 25: 275–288
2. De Santis A, Laiacona M, Barbarotto R, Basso A, Villani R, Spagnoli D, Capitani E (1989) Neuropsychological outcome of patients operated upon for an intracranial aneurysm. Analysis of general prognostic factor and of the effects of the location of the aneurysm. J Neurol Neurosurg Psychiatry 52: 1123–1140
3. Hütter BO, Gilsbach JM (1992) Cognitive deficits after rupture and early repair of anterior communicating artery aneurysms. Acta Neurochir (Wien) 116: 6–13
4. Hütter BO, Gilsbach JM (1993) Which neuropsychological defictis are hidden behind a good outcome (Glasgow = I) after aneurysmal subarachnoid hemorrhage? Neurosurgery 33: 999–1006
5. Hütter BO, Kreitschmann-Andermahr I, Gilsbach JM (2001) Quality of life after aneurysmal subarachnoid haemorrhage. J Neurosurg 94: 241–250
6. Kaku Y, Yonekawa Y, Tsukahara T, Kazekawa K (1992) Superselective intra-arterial infusion of papaverine for the treatment of cerebral vasospasm after subarachnoid hemorrhage. J Neurosurg 77: 842–847
7. Krayenbühl N, Hegner T, Yonekawa Y, Keller E (2001) Cerebral vasospasm after subarachnoid hemorrhage: hypertensive hypervolemic hemodilution (triple-H) therapy according to new systemic hemodynamic parameters. Acta Neurochir. (Suppl), in press
8. Lanzino G, Kassell NF, Germanson TP, Kongable GL, Truskowski LL, Torner JC, Jane JA, and the Participants (1996) Age and outcome after aneurysmal subarachnoid hemorrhage: why do older patients fare worse? J Neurosurg 85: 410–418
9. Ljunggren B, Sonesson B, Säveland H, Brandt L (1985) Cognitive impairment and adjustment in patients without neurological deficits after aneurysmal SAH and early operation. J Neurosurg 62: 673–679
10. Maurice-Wiliams RS, Wilison JR, Hatfield R (1991) The cognitive and psychological sequelae of uncomplicated aneurysm surgery. J Neurol Neurosurg Psychiatry 54: 335–340
11. McKenna P, Wilison JR, Lowe D, Neil-Dwyer G (1989) Cognitive outcome and quality of life one year after subarachnoid hemorrhage. Neurosurgery 24: 361–367
12. Ogden JA, Mee EW, Henning M (1993) A prospective study of impairment of cognition and memory and recovery after subarachnoid hemorrhage. Neurosurgery 33: 572–587
13. Tidswell P, Dias PS, Sagar HJ, Mayes AR, Battersby RDE (1995) Cognitive outcome after aneurysm rupture: relationship to aneurysm site and perioperative complications. Neurology 45: 875–882
14. Vilkki J (1985) Amnesic syndromes after surgery of anterior communicating artery aneurysms. Cortex 21: 431–444
15. Volpe BT, Hirst (1983) Amnesia following the rupture and repair of an anterior communicating artery aneurysm. J Neurol Neurosurg Psychiatry 46: 704–709

Correspondence: M. Bjeljac, M.D., Department of Neurosurgery, University Hospital, Frauenklinikstrasse 10, CH-8091 Zurich, Switzerland.

Acta Neurochir (2002) [Suppl] 82: 87–92

New Methods for Monitoring Cerebral Oxygenation and Hemodynamics in Patients with Subarachnoid Hemorrhage

E. Keller[1], **A. Nadler**[2], **H.-G. Imhof**[1], **P. Niederer**[2], **P. Roth**[1], and **Y. Yonekawa**[1]

[1] Department of Neurosurgery, University of Zurich, Zurich, Switzerland
[2] Department of Biomedicine, University of Zurich, Zurich, Switzerland

Summary

Radiographic cerebral vasospasm (CVS) after subarachnoid hemorrhage (SAH) do not reflect cerebral hemodynamics and oxygenation and may occur in the absence of clinical deficit and vice-versa. This report is to describe preliminary findings in further development of a non invasive method to estimate regional cerebral oxygenation and perfusion. Measurements were performed with a technique combining near infrared spectroscopy (NIRS) and indocyaningreen (ICG) dye dilution. Successful data analysis has been performed based on the decomposition in pulsatile and non-pulsatile components of NIRS absorption data collected before and during the passage of ICG through the vascular bed under the NIRS-detector. First measurements in patients with CVS suggest that the technique could become a powerful tool in the detection and treatment of CVS. This non invasive technique can be done at the bedside, it seems to be safe, easy to perform and less time-consuming compared to conventional techniques.

The influence of extracerebral bone and surface tissue on cerebral NIRS signal has not been clarified yet. Therefore a new subdural NIRS probe has been developed, which gives the opportunity to measure directly the concentration of the chromophores in the brain without the influence of extracerebral contamination. In future comparative measurements with conventional NIRS probes on the scalp will allow to quantify and eliminate extracerebral contamination from the NIRS signal.

Keywords: Subarachnoid hemorrhage; cerebral blood flow; indocyaningreen; near infrared spectroscopy.

Introduction

Discrepancies between angiographic cerebral vasospasm (CVS), transcranial Doppler (TCD) blood flow velocities (Vm) and delayed cerebral ischemic deficits (DID) after subarachnoid hemorrhage (SAH) are documented in the literature [19, 29]. Angiographic CVS fails to reflect cerebral perfusion and oxygenation patterns, responsible for DID due to CVS. The search

of an easy, safe and reliable method to detect and control treatment of clinically relevant CVS is still a matter of investigation.

The aim of the present project is to develop a new method to estimate regional cerebral oxygen patterns, cerebral blood volume (CBV) and cerebral blood flow (CBF) by a combination of near infrared spectroscopy (NIRS) and indocyaningreen (ICG) dye dilution.

The reliability of NIRS in the adult head may be restricted by contamination of the cerebral NIRS signal with blood from extracerebral tissue. Therefore a new subdural NIRS probe has been developed, which gives the opportunity to measure directly the concentration of the chromophores in the brain without the influence of extracerebral contamination.

Material and Methods

Patient Population and Treatment

The study was approved by the Ethics Committee of the University of Zurich (E-016/99). 10 patients with aneurysmal SAH were prospectively studied. TCD- and NIRS measurements were obtained routinely every 24 hours. Surgery to clip the ruptured aneurysm was performed as soon as scheduling permitted (mean day 2). Triple-H therapy (hypertensive hypervolemic hemodilution) was induced if transcranial doppler (TCD) blood flow velocities increased (Vm middle cerebral artery > 120 cm/sec or increase > 30 cm/sec within 24 hours) and/or the patient developed deficits from CVS. Patients with allergies were excluded. If patients with DID did not improve or worsened instead of triple-H therapy, after exclusion of hypoxia, electrolyte imbalance and hydrocephalus, angiography and treatment with percutaneous angioplasty and/or superselective papaverine infusion into the vasospastic vessels were performed. Symptomatic CVS, resistant or reoccurring after angioplasty and papaverine were treated with barbiturate coma and/or hypothermia according to our standardized treatment regimen.

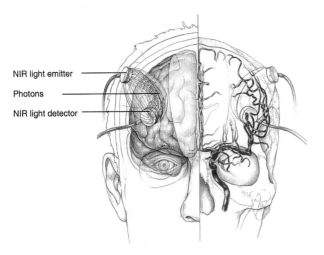

Fig. 1. Conventional NIRS technique: 2 pairs of NIRS sensors are placed bilaterally on the forehead, emitter and detector 5 cm apart. Light grey shaded area: anterior cerebral artery (ACA) territory. Dark grey shaded area: middle cerebral artery (MCA) territory

Instrumentation: NIRS with Optodes on the Scalp

4 near infrared spectroscopy (NIRS) optodes were placed bilaterally on the forehead, 2 emitters and 2 detectors, 5 cm apart (Fig. 1). OD changes were recorded by the NIRS-system (Oxymon-Systems, Nijmegen, Netherlands, 10 Hz sampling frequency, 769, 850, 905 nm). Central venous injections of 25 mg ICG (12.5 mg/1 ml aqua dest.) were performed. The appearance of ICG in the optical field and dye dilution curves were recorded.

Instrumentation: NIRS with Optodes Placed in the Subdural Space

A conventional subdural probe for ICP monitoring (NMT Neurosciences) has been supplied with a 2 mm thick and 25 cm long NIRS probe consisting of two fiber bundles (Fig. 2). Both fiber bundles are terminated with a 90-degree prism, the first one to couple the infrared light into the tissue and the second one to couple it back into the fibers (Fig. 3). The distance between the two prisms is 3.5 cm.

Signal Processing

Data analysis was performed separating the signals in the arterial and venous compartments in the optical segment detected by NIRS

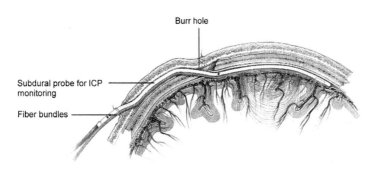

Fig. 2. Combined subdural ICP-NIRS probe: inserted through a burr hole in the skull the probe gives direct access to the brain and elimination of extracranial contamination is gained

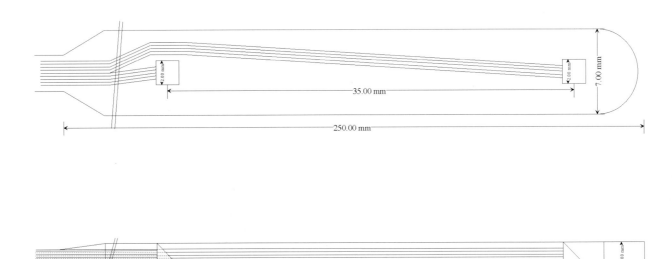

Fig. 3. NIRS subdural probe: 25 cm long and 2 mm thick. Two fiber bundles and two prisms are embedded in soft silicone. The prisms are separated by 3.5 cm

Subdural ICP-NIRS probe

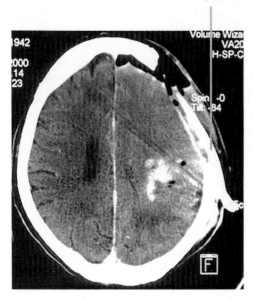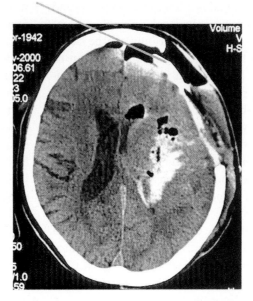

Fig. 4. CT scan of a patient with intracerebral hemorrhage after surgical hematoma evacuation. The ICP-NIRS probe is positioned subdural over the left hemisphere

[31]. The different compartments can be identified by their special changes in blood volume. The arterial blood volume pulsates with systole and diastole. As in pulse oximetry, these pulsations are used to identify the arterial compartment of the optical segment. Using digital bandpass filters the arterial contribution to the ICG indicator dilution curve is qualitatively identified. The cumulative NIRS signal obtained over the cortex can be quantified as $C_{ICG}^{Tissue} = \int i(t) - o(t)$, whereas $i(t)$ represents the inlet and $o(t)$ the outlet of the system. The convolution integral $o(t) = i(t - u) * g(u)$ describes the relationship between input and output function, whereas $g(u)$ is also termed "transport function" in the context of indicator dilution theory [1]. By iterative approximation the arterial contribution (input function) and the venous contribution (output function) to the ICG indicator dilution curve is quantified. The cerebral blood volume (CBV) is defined as the volume fraction of blood in cerebral tissue. As ICG remains strictly intravascular CBV can be calculated from $CBV = C_{ICG}^{Tissue}(t)/C_{ICG}^{Blood}(t)$, whereas C_{ICG}^{Tissue} is the accumulation of ICG in the examined brain tissue and C_{ICG}^{Blood} the concentration of ICG in the blood. CBF is calculated from CBV divided by the corresponding mtt_{ICG}.

Results

NIRS with Optodes on the Scalp

In 10 patients 63 measurements were obtained. No complications associated with the measurement method were observed. Filtering the data showed that the amplitude of pulsatile absorption changes was high enough for further signal processing in 52 measurements. The mean value for mtt_{ICG} was 8.7 sec (range 3.8 to 12.2 sec) for the right hemisphere. For the left hemisphere the mean value for mtt_{ICG} was 8.2 sec (5 to 13.8 sec). 32 pairs of repeated measurements were performed within 15 mins under stable clinical conditions (unchanged intracranial pressure, mean arterial blood pressure and $PaCO_2$). The correlation of repeated measurements was for mtt_{ICG} 0.82.

NIRS with Optodes Placed in the Subdural Space

The prototype of the subdural NIRS probe could be successfully inserted in a first patient with intracerebral hemorrhage after surgical hematoma evacuation (Fig. 4). 16 simultaneous measurements with conventional NIRS (optodes placed on the skin) and the subdural NIRS probe were performed. Signal strength obtained with the subdural probe was better and mtt_{ICG} were shorter than mtt_{ICG} obtained with conventional NIRS (mean values 6.0 sec. to 4.8 sec.).

Discussion

After SAH the complex changes of cerebral hemodynamics and oxygenation pattern with the development of CVS are underestimated if TCD-monitoring and angiography are considered singularly. The role of TCD in predicting symptomatic CVS is limited to the cases in whom very high Vm are detected [29]. Moreover, to control the treatment of CVS, TCD values are influenced by triple-H therapy [20]. Discrepancies between radiographic findings and DID may depend on the relationship between local cerebral oxygen-requirement and -delivery, which only can be determined if CBF and cerebral oxygen extraction can be estimated. Low CBF has been identified as independent predictor of poor outcome after SAH [18]. Nevertheless the established methods for bedside measurement of CBF with inert tracers such as the nitrous oxide dilution method or the ^{133}Xenon dilution technique are technically difficult and time consuming [16, 25]. Stable xenon-enhanced computed tomography, positron emission tomography and magnetic resonance spectroscopy are powerful research tools, but require that the patient be transported, which carries a potentially high risk. Recently a new double indicator dilution technique for bedside monitoring of CBF in combination with jugular bulb oximetry became available [14, 30]. Nevertheless first examinations in patients with SAH showed that the sensitivity of the new method to detect CVS may be limited by the technique measuring global CBF values [11]. Techniques, based on jugular bulb catheters, represent only global cerebral oxygenation and perfusion. A decrease of the jugular bulb oxygen saturation (SjvO$_2$) may be useful only in detecting severe proximal CVS, leading to significant reduction of hemispheric blood flow. The sensitivity of SjvO$_2$ to detect smaller ischemic areas secondary to CVS of single vessels is limited [11]. In cases of distal arterial narrowing, techniques measuring regional values of local cortical perfusion, representing selected vascular territories, may be more sensitive. Monitoring of partial pressure of brain tissue oxygen (PbtO$_2$) is suitable to detect focal changes in cerebral oxygenation pattern [10]. PbtO$_2$-monitoring, nevertheless, using intraparenchymatous brain catheters is an invasive method, giving accurate results only in sedated patients. Moreover CVS may occur in different vascular territories not observed with the PbtO$_2$-monitoring. The limitations of the available techniques encourage to develop a practical method for measuring regional cerebral perfusion and oxygen metabolism noninvasively in different vascular territories.

NIRS with Optodes on the Scalp

The NIRS measurement of CBF is based upon the finding that light in the near infrared region penetrates biological tissue and is absorbed differently by the chromophores Hb$_{oxy}$, Hb$_{desoxy}$, and ICG [13]. Edwards *et al.* proposed the measurement of CBF by monitoring changes in Hb$_{oxy}$ in response to changes in inspired oxygen as a tracer [6, 8]. The peripheral concentration of the tracer is measured using pulse oximetry and the accumulation of tracer in the brain is measured by NIRS. This technique showed a good correlation with the Xenon^{133} dilution method in neonates [2, 28]. In animal experiments and in adults coefficients of variation of repeated measurements were high and the O$_2$-dilution method showed poor correlation with established methods [7, 9, 24]. Colacino *et al.* reported the injection of ICG into the carotid artery in ducks and analysed the clearance curve of the dye by NIRS [4]. The combination of NIRS and dye dilution with ICG in order to estimate CBF has been described in adults and newborn infants undergoing cardiopulmonary bypass [27, 3]. The input signal of the head, nevertheless, the arterial concentration of the tracer in all studies was quantified invasively by an arterial fiberoptic-catheter placed in the aorta, or in the arterial line of the cardiopulmonary bypass circuit [22]. The objective of our project is to develop a strictly non invasive method. Therefore, a completely new approach to analyze the ICG dilution curves was performed. The cumulative signal recorded by NIRS is separated into the arterial and venous compartments with digital bandpass filters. The different compartments are identified by their special changes in blood volume [31]. This signal processing allows quantifying the input function and to estimate mt$_{tICG}$, CBV and CBF without any further catheter installations.

NIRS with Optodes Placed in the Subdural Space

The effects of bone and surface tissue blood flow on transcutaneous reflectance-mode NIRS has been extensively discussed in clinical investigations [7, 17, 23, 26, 32]. The effect of discrete anatomical layers has been modeled. Using a simple Monte Carlo simulation of the adult head comprising two concentric spheres of differing media, Hiraoka *et al.* calculated that the pathlength of NIR light in cerebral tissue was 40–55% of the total pathlength [12]. Studying the effect of the CSF layer in a more complex model Cui *et al.* found that at an emitter-detector separation of 5.0 cm, 55% of the NIR light pathlength was in the scalp and skull, 20% in the CSF and only 15% of the NIR pathlength was in the cerebral cortex [5]. Because CSF has low scattering and absorption coefficients, the authors postulated that the CSF is acting as a "channel" for the light. On the other hand, first measurements with the transcutaneous NIRS ICG dilution technique before and after superselective papaverine infusion into vasospastic vessels indicate, that data obtained by the NIRS ICG dye dilution technique at least represent a significant contribution from the intracerebral vessels [15]. Most attempts to subtract extracerebral contamination involve spatial resolved spectroscopy (SRS) [21]. Nevertheless interindividual variability of anatomical structures (bone thickness, extracerebral vasculature, liquor space, etc.) may restrict the reliability of SRS. In the present project the prototype of a subdural NIRS probe could be developed and inserted in a first patient. The new subdural NIRS probe will give the opportunity to measure directly the concentration of the chromophores in the cortex without the influence of extracerebral tissue. To calculate the contribution of extracerebral contamination comparative measurements have been performed alternatively with conventional NIRS probes on the scalp. Mtt_{ICG} obtained with the subdural probe were shorter than those obtained with transcutaneous NIRS. This corresponds with Doppler examinations and cerebral angiography findings showing that transit times of contrast materials are longer in the extracerebral vasculature than in the brain vessels. For NIRS a conventional subdural probe for ICP monitoring has been supplied with fiber bundles. Intracranial pressure (ICP) monitoring with a subdural probe is a well-established technique in Neurocritical Care to detect and treat intracranial hypertension. Combined monitoring of ICP and NIRS will be of special clinical value in patients with severe head trauma and subarachnoid hemorrhage, already installed with subdural ICP-probes for treatment of intracranial hypertension and being especially at risk for secondary ischemic brain damage.

In conclusion our preliminary studies suggest that conventional NIRS extended with the ICG dye dilution technique is safe and easy to perform. Successful data analysis has been performed based on the decomposition in pulsatile and non-pulsatile components of the NIRS absorption data.

The technique could be a powerful tool in detection and treatment of CVS causing DID.

Validation of the method in a larger set of patients with H_2O-PET measurements are needed.

The new combined subdural ICP-NIRS probe will give the opportunity to measure directly the concentration of the chromophores in the brain without the influence of extracerebral tissue. Combined monitoring of ICP and NIRS will be of special clinical value in critically ill patients with treatment of intracranial hypertension.

References

1. Bassingthwaighte JB (1967) Circulatory transport and the convolution integral. Mayo Clin Proc 42: 137–154
2. Bucher HU, Edwards AD, Lipp AE, Duc G (1993) Comparison between near infrared spectroscopy and 133Xenon clearance for estimation of cerebral blood flow in critically ill preterm infants. Pediatr Res 33: 56–60
3. Chow G, Roberts IG, Fallon P, Onoe M, Lloyd-Thomas A, Elliott MJ, Edwards AD, Kirkham FJ (1997) The relation between arterial oxygen tension and cerebral blood flow during cardiopulmonary bypass. Eur J Cardiothorac Surg 11: 633–639
4. Colacino JM, Grubb B, Jobsis FF (1981) Infrared technique for cerebral blood flow: Comparison with 133Xenon clearance. Neurol Res 3: 17–31
5. Cui W, Kumar C, Chance B (1991) Experimental study of migration depth for the photons measured at sample surface. Proc Soc Photooptival Instrumentation Eng 1431: 180–191
6. Edwards AD, Wyatt JS, Richardson C, Delpy D, Cope M, Reynolds EO (1988) Cotside measurement of cerebral blood flow in ill newborn infants by near infrared spectroscopy. Lancet 2: 770–771
7. Elwell CE, Cope M, Edwards AD, Wyatt JS, Delpy DT, Reynolds EOR (1994) Quantification of adult cerebral hemodynamics by near-infrared spectroscopy. J Appl Physiol 77: 2753–2760
8. Elwell CE, Owen-Reece H, Cope M, Edwards AD, Wyatt JS, Reynolds EO, Delpy DT (1994) Measurement of changes in cerebral haemodynamics during inspiration and exspiration using near infrared spectroscopy. Adv Exp Med Biol 345: 619–624
9. Elwell CE, Cope M, Edwards AD, Wyatt JS, Reynolds EOR, Delpy DT (1992) Oxygen Transport to Tissue XIV, vol. 317. In: Erdmann W, Bruley DF (eds) Plenum Press, New York, pp 235–245
10. Fandino J, Stocker R, Prokop S, Imhof HG (1999) Correlation between jugular bulb oxygen saturation and partial pressure of brain tissue oxygen during CO2 and O2 reactivity tests in severely head-injured patients. Acta Neurochir (Wien) 141: 825–834
11. Hegner T, Krayenbühl N, Hefti M, Yonekawa Y, Keller E (2001) Bedside monitoring of cerebral blood flow in subarachnoid hemorrhage. Acta Neurochir (Wien) in press
12. Hiraoka M, Firbank M, Essenpreis M, Cope M, Arridge SR, van der Zee P, Delpy DT (1993) A Monte Carlo investigation of optical pathlength in inhomogenous tissue and its application to near-infrared spectroscopy. Phys Med Biol 38: 1859–1876
13. Jöbsis FF (1977) Noninvasive, infrared monitoring of cerebral and myocardial oxygen sufficiency and circulatory parameters. Science 198: 1264–1267
14. Keller E, Wietasch G, Ringleb P, Scholz M, Schwarz S, Stingele R, Schwab S, Hanley D, Hache W (2000) Bedside monitoring of cerebral blood flow in patients with acute hemispheric stroke. Crit Care Med 28: 511–516
15. Keller E, Wolf M, Martin M, Fandino J, Roth P, Yonekawa Y (2001) Estimation of cerebral oxygenation and hemodynamics in cerebral vasospasm using indocyaningreen (ICG) dye dilution and near infrared spectroscopy (NIRS). A case report. J Neurosurg Anethesiol 13: 43–48

16. Kety SS, Schmidt CF (1945) The determination of cerebral blood flow in man by the use of nitrous oxide in low concentrations. Am J Physiol 143: 53

17. Kirkpatrick PJ, Smielewski P, Whitfield PC, Czosnyka M, Menon D, Pickard JD (1995) An observational study of near-infrared spectroscopy during carotid endarterectomy. J Neurosurg 82: 756–763

18. Lennihan L, Mayer SA, Fink ME, Beckford A, Paik MC, Zahng H, Wu Y, Kelbanoff LM, Raps EC, Solomon RA (2000) Effect of hypervolemic therapy on cerebral blood flow after subarachnoid hemorrhage: a randomized controlled trial. Stroke 31: 383–391

19. Lindegaard KF (1999) The role of transcranial Doppler in the management of patients with subarachnoid hemorrhage – a review. Acta Neurochir (Wien) 72: 59–71

20. Manno EM, Gress DR, Schwamm LH, Diringer MN, Ogilvy CS (1998) Effects of induced hypertension on transcranial Doppler ultrasound velocities in patients after subarachnoid hemorrhage. Stroke 29: 422–428

21. Matcher SJ, Kirkpatrick P, Nahid K, Cope M, Delpy DT (1995) Absolute quantification methods in tissue near infrared spectroscopy. SPIE 2389: 486–495

22. McCormick PW, Stewart M, Goetting MG, Dujovny M, Lewis G, Ausman JI (1991) Noninvasive cerebral optical spectroscopy for monitoring cerebral oxygen delivery and hemodynamics. Crit Care Med 19: 89–97

23. McCormick PW, Stewart M, Lewis G, Dujovny M, Ausman JI (1992) Intracerebral penetration of infrared light. Technical note. J Neurosurg 76: 315–318

24. Newton CR, Wilson DA, Gunnoe E, Wagner B, Cope M, Traystman RJ (1997) Measurement of cerebral blood flow in dogs with near infrared spectroscopy in the reflectance mode is invalid. J Cereb Blood Flow Metab 17: 695–703

25. Obrist WD, Thompson HK, Wang HS, Wilkinson WE (1975) Regional cerebral blood flow estimated by 133-xenon inhalation. Stroke 6: 245–256

26. Owen-Reece H, Elwell CE, Wyatt JS, Delpy DT (1996) The effect of scalp ischemia on measurement of cerebral blood volume by near-infrared spectroscopy. Physiol Meas 17: 279–286

27. Roberts I, Fallon P, Kirkham FJ, Loyd-Thomas A, Cooper C, Maynard R, Elliot M, Edwards AD (1993) Estimation of cerebral blood flow with near infrared spectroscopy and indocyanine green. Lancet 342: 1425

28. Skov L, Pryds O, Greisen G (1991) Estimating cerebral blood flow in newborn infants: Comparison of near infrared spectroscopy and 133Xe clearance. Pediatr Res 30: 570–573

29. Vora YY, Suarez-Almazor M, Steinke DE, Martin ML, Findlay JM (1999) Role of transcranial Doppler monitoring in the diagnosis of cerebral vasospasm after subarachnoid hemorrhage. Neurosurgery 44: 1237–1248

30. Wietasch GJK, Mielck F, Scholz M, von Spiegel T, Stephan H, Hoeft A (2000) Bedside assessment of cerebral blood flow by double-indicator dilution technique. Anesthesiology 92: 367–375

31. Wolf M, Duc G, Keel M, Niederer P, von Siebenthal K, Bucher HU (1997) Continuous noninvasive measurement of cerebral arterial and venous oxygen saturation at the bedside in mechanically ventilated neonates. Crit Care Med 25: 1579–1582

32. Young AER, Germon TJ, Barnett NJ, Manara AR, Nelson RJ (2000) Behaviour of near-infrared light in the adult human head: Implications for clinical near-infrared spectroscopy. Br J Anaesth 84: 38–42

Correspondence: Emanuela Keller, M.D., Department of Neurosurgery, University Hospital, Frauenklinikstrasse 10, 8091 Zurich, Switzerland.

Acta Neurochir (2002) [Suppl] 82: 93–98
© Springer-Verlag 2002

Role of Hypothermia in the Management of Severe Cases of Subarachnoid Hemorrhage

N. Yasui[1], S. Kawamura[1], A. Suzuki[1], H. Hadeishi[1], and J. Hatazawa[2]

[1] Department of Surgical Neurology, Research Institute for Brain and Blood Vessels, Akita, Japan
[2] Department of Neuroradiology, Research Institute for Brain and Blood Vessels, Akita, Japan

Summary

Mild hypothermia is thought to have a brain protective effect to pathophysiological conditions, which are caused by severe brain damage including brain injury and cerebral stroke. In this paper, general aspects of this treatment as history, pathophysiological effect, and problems are summarized. Also, the clinical effects of hypothermic therapy for a subarachnoid hemorrhage are reviewed. Main targets of the therapy for this disease are severe primary brain damage caused by the attack itself and secondary ischemic brain damage after delayed vasospasm. But even now, there are no fully established data about the effect of hypothermia at such conditions after subarachnoid hemorrhage. The results of our study of cerebral blood flow and cerebral oxygen metabolism using positron emission tomography are presented to show the physiological effect of hypothermia on human brain after severe brain damage caused by subarachnoid hemorrhage.

In conclusion, effect of hypothermia on subarachnoid hemorrhage is not confirmed yet and reported data is limited, so that additional studies, especially controlled studies, would be recommended.

Keywords: Brain protection; mild hypothermia; subarachnoid hemorrhage; primary brain damage.

Introduction

Mild hypothermia is expected to have a brain protective effect on pathophysiological conditions after subarachnoid hemorrhage [12, 14, 16, 28]. Main targets of this therapy are severe primary brain damage caused by the attack itself and secondary ischemic brain damage after delayed vasospasm. But till now, there are no confirmed data about the effect of hypothermia on subarachnoid hemorrhage. In this paper, the results of several studies on mild hypothermia, especially after subarachnoid hemorrhage are reviewed and data including the results of cerebral blood flow (CBF) and cerebral oxygen metabolism (CMRO$_2$) [15, 16] are presented to give an overview of the present status of hypothermic therapy after subarachnoid hemorrhage.

Effects of Mild Hypothermia

The brain protective effect of hypothermia has been well known for a long time [9, 21, 30], and it has been applied to cardiac surgery and cerebral aneurysm surgery to protect the brain from blood standstill during the operation. Deep hypothermia lowering the body temperature to less than 30 degrees was done in the 1950's [3, 4], but maintenance of the low temperature and management of the patient were complicated by that method. There had been serious general complications connected with this method for a long time so that it was rarely performed as a treatment method for brain disease.

This treatment method came to the limelight again when Busto reported in 1987 [5] that brain protective effect was provided by mild hypothermia that lowers the brain temperature by only a few degrees. Serious general complications, which are problems of deep hypothermia, were reduced with mild hypothermia, and expansion of the clinical application range was possible and patient management became more easy. As a result, the brain protective effect of mild hypothermia was used in severe head injury [22, 23, 29] and cerebral apoplexy [26], and became an accepted treatment modality. However, a treatment effect of mild hypothermia has still not been established for severe cases of cerebral stroke such as subarachnoid hemorrhage, cerebral infarction and intracerebral hemorrhage.

Although the effects of hypothermia have been investigated extensively, particularly in ischemic brain damage, the mechanisms associated with therapeutic hypothermia are not fully understood. Hypothermic neuroprotection may be related to suppression of major biochemical processes such as cerebral metabolism and excitatory neurotransmitter release [6, 10, 23], as well as inhibition of accumulation of lipid peroxidation products and free radical generation [2]. Both CBF and $CMRO_2$ decrease during hypothermia [10, 16]. The $CMRO_2$ reduction can result in a decrease in energy demand by the brain. The cerebral protective effects of hypothermia may also be a function of economizing CBF with the prevention of postischemic hyper- and hypoperfusion, blood-brain barrier disruption, and formation of brain edema [8, 13]. Attenuation of brain acidosis and inflammatory responses may also be potential mechanisms [18, 31]. In reality, numerous mechanisms are probably responsible for decreasing the intracranial pressure and the protective effects of hypothermia.

The following conditions are expected to have a brain protective effect of hypothermia in a patient of subarachnoid hemorrhage. Main targets of this therapy are severe primary brain damage caused by bleeding attack itself and secondary ischemic brain damage after delayed vasospasm.

Problems of Hypothermia

A brain protective effect, as mentioned above in hypothermia therapy, is expected in severe brain disease. However, as for hypothermia, there are many problems that should be solved in clinical practice because a lot of problems exist in this treatment. Somehow, this method is very complicated and very difficult in the management of patients.

To maintain general circulatory conditions, oxygen delivery should be kept at more than 800 ml/min. monitored by Swan-Ganz Catheter, during hypothermia in order to get a useful effect. In addition, the end-expiratory carbon dioxide concentration has to be maintained at more than 32–38 mmHg, arterial carbon dioxide concentration at more than 34–38 mmHg, oxygen saturation at more than 98%, and hemoglobin at more than 12 gr/dl as an index of oxygen delivery [11]. Blood sugar level has to be maintained at less than 180 mg/dl and do maintenance more than 3.0 g/dl with an aim with serum albumin.

Furthermore, various general complications as described in the following may occur, and prevention and treatment of them are very important in order not to endanger an effect of this treatment method. In particular, the most frequent and serious complication is infectious disease such as pneumonia [6]. Other complications that may happen when performing hypothermia therapy are cardiovascular problems of hemodynamic instability due to systemic hypotension and cardiac arrhythmias, suppression of immunity, electrolyte imbalance especially hypopotassemia, coagulopathy, multi-organ failure etc [7, 19, 21]. Even if experimental studies prove a brain protective effect of the hypothermia therapy, these complications may be detrimental to this treatment method.

Hypothermia for Primary Brain Damage after Subarachnoid Hemorrhage

Rupture of cerebral aneurysm, subarachnoid haemorrhage, intracerebral hematoma, intra-ventricular hematoma, and rarely subdural hematoma cause primary brain damage. The damage of a brain by a hematoma itself is mainly caused by intracerebral hematoma, but subarachnoid hematoma hits a brain directly and can be damaged.

Intracranial pressure suddenly rises markedly at aneurysm rupture, and therefore cerebral circulation in the whole brain is disturbed [27]. If cerebral circulation is reinstated within a few minutes, brain damage would be limited or even nil. However, if duration of the cerebral ischemia is longer, resulting brain injury is more extensive and serious. In addition, when cerebral circulation recovers in such a severe case, it is accompanied by reperfusion injury and may reinforce the brain damage [1]. In a patient with severe subarachnoid hemorrhage, this ischemic brain damage occurs in addition to the direct brain damage caused by a hematoma.

Mild hypothermia has a brain protective effect and decreases intracranial pressure in case of cerebral ischemia caused by severe subarachnoid hemorrhage. Kubo *et al.* [17] applied hypothermia treatment for 48 hours in severe cases of subarachnoid hemorrhage, but did not register among effectiveness. When patient condition was aggravated during the rewarming period, warming was stopped and the patient was cooled again with or without barbiturate therapy, but a good result was not achieved. On the other hand, Park [28] reported 17 cases of severe subarachnoid hemorrhage treated with hypothermia therapy more than 4 days after neck clipping having a comparatively good result. However, these reports represent only limited experience and no controlled trial, so additional controlled studies would be recommended.

Hypothermia for Delayed Cerebral Vasospasm

Delayed cerebral vasospasm following subarachnoid hemorrhage frequently occurred between day 4 and 14 and is one of the main causes for neurological deterioration of the patient. Delayed vasospasm decreases CBF. If CBF level drops below the ischemic threshold, cerebral infarction occurs. Various kinds of treatment may be applied for delayed vasospasm; prevention and treatment methods are not currently established. A case of cerebral infarction caused by delayed vasospasm is known even after various kinds of treatment were performed extensively. An effective treatment method for such a case that caused extensive cerebral infarction by advanced delayed vasospasm does not exist still now. For patients who suffered such serious delayed vasospasm, there are some reports with mild hypothermia being chosen to reduce brain damage [12, 14, 20, 28].

From hypothermia treatment a brain protective effect for cerebral ischemia by delayed vasospasm can be expected. However, hypothermia cannot prevent and reduce vasospasm, and narrowing of arterial diameter is extended until time of rewarming. As a result, delayed vasospasm which did prolong at the time of rewarming causes cerebral ischemia and brain edema increases it rapidly and causes brain damage. Therefore there are many reports that hypothermia does not have a clinical effect for delayed vasospasm [12, 17]. Brain damage occurring during rewarming, may result from systemic hypotension by general vasodilatation, increased metabolism as a rebound phenomenon, and increased intracranial pressure [32]. However, Kawai et al. [14] reported that brain damage in rewarming is caused by problems of the rewarming method. In particular, speed of rewarming is most important. If temperature of the patient is elevated by 0.5 to 1 degree over 24 hours, aggravation of the patient will not occur [25].

Other problems of hypothermia for delayed vasospasm include prolongation of the treatment period [12, 14, 20, 28]. Hypothermia therapy would continue more than 7 days, even if started when cerebral ischemia by delayed vasospasm appeared. It is easy to ac-

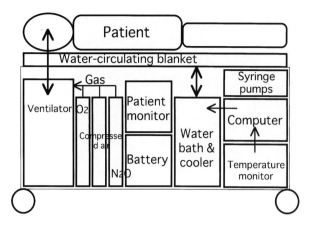

Fig. 1. Hypothermia bed system for patients with stroke

company the general complication to continue hypothermia for long period, but this frequently results in deterioration of the patient. The hypothermia therapy for delayed vasospasm still includes lots of serious problems, and these should be solved in the future.

Results of Mild Hypothermia for Severe Subarachnoid Hemorrhage and Effect on Cerebral Blood Flow and Oxygen Metabolism

Our experience with mild hypothermia for subarachnoid hemorrhage is briefly summarized here because most of the data has already been published in other journals [15, 16].

When we started hypothermia therapy, we constructed a hypothermia system bed designed for patients with stroke (Fig. 1) [15]. The system bed contained all necessary equipment including a respirator, a cooling unit, physiological monitors, and a storage battery. Surface cooling of the patients was performed using water-circulating blankets, and core temperature was maintained based on bladder temperature and a feedback computer program. During hypothermia therapy, patient transfer and radiological examination including computed tomography, and single photon and positron emission tomography (PET) could be easily and safely performed (Fig. 2). Differences between the measured bladder temperature and the target temperature were approximately $\pm 0.1\,^{\circ}C$. The proposed hypothermia system bed may be useful for serial radiological examination of patients with stroke including severe subarachnoid hemorrhage.

Mild hypothermia was indicated for aneurysmal subarachnoid hemorrhage patients who satisfied the

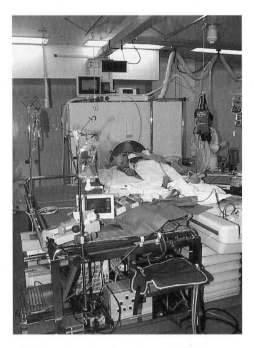

Fig. 2. Photograph showing patient during measurement of positron emission tomography

Table 1. *Hypothermic Therapy for Subarachnoid Hemorrhage ('00, 7)*

Case	Age/sex	AN	ICH	GCS (WFNS)	Barthel index
1	37/F	lt ICA	frontal	4 (5)	85 (16 mo)
2	49/M	lt SCA-BA	–	8 (4)	100 (10 mo)
3	54/M	rt MCA	frontal	3 (5)	60 (17 mo)
4	67/F	lt MCA	frontal	7 (4)	0 (12 mo)
5	43/M	rt MCA	–	6 (5)	0 (12 mo)
6	65/F	lt ACA	bi-frontal	4 (5)	5 (12 mo)
7	47/F	lt MCA	frontotemp.	7 (4)	0 (6 mo)

ICH Intracerebral hematoma, *GCS* Glasgow coma scale, *WFNS* universal subarachnoid hemorrhage grading scale by the World Federation of Neurosurgical Surgeons, *ICA* internal carotid artery, *SCA* superior cerebellar artery, *BA* basilar artery, *MCA* middle cerebral artery, *ACA* distal anterior cerebral artery.

following criteria: time from hemorrhage to admission of less than 6 hours; age less than 70 years old; no past-history of ischemic heart disease; level of consciousness upon admission of semi-comatose or worse, or stage IV or V according to the WFNS scale; and spontaneous respiration.

From June 1997 to July 2000, of 188 subarachnoid hemorrhage patients admitted to our hospital, seven (3.7%) satisfied the criteria for inclusion in the study and underwent hypothermic therapy. We investigated cerebral blood flow and oxygen metabolism using PET

Table 2. *PET Parameters During Hypothermic Therapy*

Case no	Ipsilateral MCA area				Contralateral MCA area			
	CBF	$CMRO_2$	OEF	CBV	CBF	$CMRO_2$	OEF	CBV
2	25	1.94	0.57	3.7	25	1.88	0.54	4.3
3	39	1.72	0.32	3.4	33	2.26	0.42	4.2
4	40	1.85	0.33	2.8	41	2.72	0.47	5.1
5	27	1.38	0.29	3.7	30	1.97	0.40	6.4
6	43	2.36	0.47*	4.7	29	2.22	0.55	3.2
7	40	1.30	0.24	3.7	36	2.62	0.51	3.0
Mean	35.7	1.76	0.37	3.7	32.3	2.28	0.48	4.4
SD	7.6	0.39	0.12	0.6	5.6	0.34	0.06	1.3

* Range = 0.28–0.60, Data represent mean value of three ROIs, *MCA* middle cerebral artery, *CBF* cerebral blood flow (mml/100 ml/min), *OEF* oxygen extraction fraction, $CMRO_2$ cerebral metabolic rate of oxygen (ml/100 ml/min), *CBV* cerebral blood volume (ml/100 ml). *SD* Standard deviation.

in 6 of the 7 patients during hypothermia (33–34 °C) with severe subarachnoid hemorrhage (Table 1). Clinical outcome was evaluated using Barthel index. Their preoperative clinical condition was WFNS scale IV in 3 cases and V in 4 cases. The patients received surface cooling postoperatively, the core temperature was lowered further to 33–34 °C over the course of approximately 48 hours, and then rewarmed over the subsequent 48 hours. They were maintained in a hypothermic state during transfer for radiological examination.

Clinical results are shown in Table 1. Cases 1 and 2 had a good surgical outcome and were able to function and live independently. Case 3 was partially dependent and could walk with assistance. Cases 4–7 were bedridden until 12 months following SAH. None of the patients died during the follow-up-period. All 7 patients had no complications which were considered to be related to the hypothermic therapy.

PET revealed a decrease in cerebral blood flow and oxygen metabolic rate. CBF was 35.7 ± 7.6 ml/100 ml/min and $CMRO_2$ was 1.76 ± 0.39 ml/100 ml/min in areas of the middle cerebral artery ipsilateral to the ruptured aneurysms, whereas these values were 32.3 ± 5.6 and 2.28 ± 0.34 ml/100 ml/min, respectively, on the contralateral side (Table 2). This represents a decrease of $35.7 \pm 14.1\%$ compared to normal CBF and $54.3 \pm 9.9\%$ compared to normal $CMRO_2$ ($p < 0.01$) in the ipsilateral areas, and decreases of $41.8 \pm 10.1\%$ and $41.2 \pm 8.6\%$, respectively, on the contralateral side (Table 3). The present results reflected the luxury perfusion state in almost all cases (Table 4) and provide the PET evidence of decreased CBF and $CMRO_2$ during hypothermia in humans.

Table 3. *% Decreases in CBF and CMRO$_2$ During Hypothermia Compared with Normal Volunteers*

Case no	Ipsilateral MCA area		Contralateral MCA area	
	CBF	CMRO$_2$	CBF	CMRO$_2$
2	55	50	55	51
3	29	55	40	42
4	28	52	26	30
5	52	64	47	49
6	22	39	48	43
7	28	66	35	32
Mean	35.7	54.3*	41.8	41.2
SD	14.1	9.9	10.4	8.6

* p < 0.01, *SD* standard deviation.

Table 4. *Perfusion State in MCA Area During Hypothermia*

Case	ICH	Ipsilateral	Contralateral
2	−	misery	misery
3	+	luxury	coupling
4	+	luxury	coupling
5	−	luxury	coupling
6	+	※	misery
7	+	luxury	misery

ICH Intracerebral hematoma.
* Luxury around ICH and misery at superior temporal area.

Conclusion

In this paper, the results of several studies on mild hypothermia in cases of subarachnoid hemorrhage are reviewed and our data including the results of CBF and CMRO$_2$, are presented to give an overview of the present status of hypothermic therapy to subarachnoid hemorrhage. This therapy mainly covers severe primary brain damage caused by the attack itself and secondary ischemic brain damage after delayed vasospasm. However, effect of hypothermia in these conditions has not been confirmed till now and reported data is limited, so that additional studies, especially controlled studies, would be recommended.

References

1. Asano T, Sano K (1977) Pathogenetic role of noreflow phenomenon in experimental subarachnoid hemorrhage in dogs. J Neurosurg 46: 454–466
2. Baiping L, Xiujuan T, Hongwei C, Qiming X, Quling G (1994) Effect of moderate hypothermia on lipid peroxidation in canine brain tissue after cardiac arrest and resuscitation. Stroke 25: 147–152
3. Bigelow WG, Callaghan JC, Hopps JA (1950) General hypothermia for experimental intracardiac surgery. Ann Surg 132: 531–537
4. Botterell EH, Lougheed WM, Scott JW, Vandewater SL (1956) Hypothermia, and interruption of carotid, or carotid and vertebral circulation, in the surgical management of intracranial aneurysms. J Neurosurg 13: 1–42
5. Busto R (1987) Small differences in intraischemic brain temperature critically determine the extent of ischemic neuronal injury. J Cereb Blood flow Metab 7: 729–738
6. Busto R, Globus MYT, Dietrich WD et al (1989) Effect of mild hypothermia on ischemia-induced release of neurotransmitter and free fatty acids in rat brain. Stroke 20: 904–910
7. Clifton G (1992) Systemic hypothermia in treatment of brain injury. J Neurotrauma [Suppl] 9: S487–495
8. Dietrich WD, Busto R, Halley M, Valdes I (1990) The importance of brain temperature in alterations of the blood-brain barrier following cerebral ischemia. J Neuropathol Exp Neurol 49: 486–497
9. Ginsberg MD et al (1992) Therapeutic modulation of brain temperature: relevance to ischemic brain injury. Cerebrovasc Brain Metab Rev 4: 189–225
10. Hagerdal M, Harp J, Siesjo BK (1975) The effect of induced hypothermia upon oxygen consumption in the rat brain. J Neurochem 24: 311–316
11. Hayashi N (1999) The brain hypothermia therapy for prevention of vegetatio after severe brain injury. Nippon Geka Gakkai Zasshi 100(7): 443–448
12. Irie K, Nakamura T, Kawai N, Nagao S (1997) Mild hyperthermia therapy in patients with severe intracranial subarachnoid hemorrhage: Effect on the occurrence of cerebral vasospasm. Proceedings of 13th Spasm Symposium in Kyoto
13. Karibe H, Chen J, Zarow GJ, Graham SH, Weinstein PR (1994) Delayed induction of mild hypothermia to reduce infarct volume after temporary middle cerebral artery occlusion in rats. J Neurosurg 80: 112–119
14. Kawai N, Ogawa T, Matsumoto Y, Irie K, Kunishio K, Nagao S (2000) The use of mild hypothermia for patients with severe vasospasm after subarachnoid hemorrhage. Proceedings of 16th Spasm Symposium in Kyoto
15. Kawamura S, Suzuki E, Suzuki A, Yasui N (1999) Hypothermia bed system for stroke patients – technical note. Neurol Med Chir (Tokyo) 39: 466–470
16. Kawamura S, Suzuki A, Hadeishi H, Yasui N, Hatazawa J (2000) Cerebral blood flow and oxygen metabolism during mild hypothermia in patients with subarachnoid hemorrhage. Acta Neurochir (Wien) 142: 1117–1122
17. Kubo Y, Suzuki M, Manase T, Miura K, Doi M, Kudo A, Sato N, Oumama S, Kuroda K, Ogawa A (1997) Cerebral hypothermia therapy on severe subarachnoid hemorrhage – effects on cerebral vasospasm. Proceedings of 13th Spasm Symposium in Kyoto
18. Laptook AR, Corbett RJT, Burns D, Sterett R (1995) Neuronal ischemic neuroprotection by modest hypothermia is associated with attenuated brain acidosis. Stroke 26: 1240–1246
19. Lawrence R (1990) Hypothermia and blood coagulation: dissociation between enzyme activity and clotting factor levels. Circulatory Shock 32: 141–152
20. Maekawa T, Tateishi A, Sadamitsu D, Kuroda Y, Soejima Y, Kashiwagi S, Yamashita T, Ito H (1994) Clinical application of mild hypothermia in neurological disorders. Minerva Anestesiol 60: 537–540
21. Maher J, Hachinski V (1993) Hypothermia as a potential treatment for cerebral ischemia. Cerebrovasc Brain Metab Rev 5: 277–300
22. Marion DW, Obrist WD, Carlier PM et al (1993) The use of moderate therapeutic hypothermia for patients with severe head injuries: a preliminary report. J Neurosurg 79: 354–362

23. Metz C, Holzschuh M, Bein T, Woertgen C, Frey A, Frey I, Taeger K, Brawanski A (1996) Moderate hypothermia in patients with severe head injury: Cerebral and extracerebral effects. J Neurosurg 85: 533–541
24. Mitani A, Kataoka K (1991) Critical levels of extracellular glutamate mediating gerbil hyppocampal delayed neuronal death during hypothermia. Neurosci 42: 661–670
25. Nakamura T, Miyamoto O, Yamagami S *et al* (1999) Influence of rewarming conditions after hypothermia in gerbils with transient forebrain ischemia. J Neurosurg 91: 114–120
26. Naritomi H, Shimizu T, Oe H *et al* (1996) Mild hypothermia therapy in acute embolic stroke: a pilot study. J Stroke Cerebrovascl Dis 6: Suppl 1 pp 193–196
27. Nornes H, Magnaes B (1972) Intracranial pressure in patients with ruptured saccular aneurysm. J Neurosurg 36: 537–547
28. Park YS, Ishikawa J (1998) Clinical result of moderate hypothermia therapy in patients with ruptured cerebral aneurysm. J pm J Neurosurg (Tokyo) 7: 71–78
29. Shiozaki T, Sugimoto H, Taneda M, Yoshida H, Iwai A, Yoshioka T, Sugimoto T (1993) Effect of mild hypothermia on uncontrollable intracranial hypertension after severe head injury. J Neurosurg 79: 363–368
30. Siebke H, Rod T, Breivik H, Lind B (1975) Survival after 40 minutes' submersion without cerebral sequelae. Lancet 1: 1275–1277
31. Toyoda T, Suzuki S, Kassell NF, Lee KS (1996) Intraischemic hypothermia attenuates neutrophil infiltration in the rat neocortex after focal ischemia-reperfusion injury. Neurosurgery 39: 1200–1205
32. Van der Linden J, Ekroth R, Lincoln C, Pugsley W, Scallan M, Tyden H (1989) Is cerebral blood flow/metabolic mismatch during rewarming a risk factor after profound hypothermic procedures in small children? Eur J Cardiothrac Surg 3: 209–215

Correspondence: N. Yasui, M.D., Department of Surgical Neurology, Research Institute for Brain and Blood Vessels, Akita, 6-10 Senshu-kubota-machi, Akita 010-0874, Japan.

Acta Neurochir (2002) [Suppl] 82: 99–103

Endovascular Aneurysm Treatment from the Neurosurgeon's Point of View

Y. Kaku

Department of Neurosurgery, Gifu University School of Medicine, Gifu, Japan

Summary

Recent advancement in microneurosurgery and interventional neuroradiology has brought us a new aspect in the treatment of cerebral aneurysms. There is now a choice of several therapeutic alternatives for the management of cerebral aneurysms. The selection of interventional neuroradiologic techniques with GDC therefore requires consideration of neurosurgical techniques, just as the selection of neurosurgical treatment requires an analysis of endovascular alternatives. The decision for treatment of an individual patient should be based on objective selection of the safest and the most effective treatment. It is self-evident that the primary consideration in the selection process must be the immediate and long-term welfare of the individual patient, rather than the physician's preference for any specific treatment modality.

Although GDC embolization has been successful in preventing acute subsequent bleeding of aneurysms, incomplete endovascular occlusion of aneurysm leaves the patient at risk for future expansion and future subarachnoid hemorrhage. With this limitation in mind, patients need to be very carefully chosen for GDC embolization. Endovascular treatment of intracranial aneurysms with GDCs has thus been limited to adjuvant or palliative indications for many patients.

Keywords: Cerebral aneurysm; direct surgery; endovascular treatment; GDC.

Introduction

Endovascular embolization using GDCs for complicated intracranial aneurysms has become widely accepted as an alternative to direct surgery. There is now a choice of therapeutic alternatives for the management of cerebral aneurysms [2, 6, 8]. The decision for treatment of an individual patient should be based on objective selection of the safest and the most effective treatment. In addition, less invasive and cost effective treatment should be chosen. In this article, the endovascular treatment for cerebral aneurysms with GDCs in comparison with direct surgical treatment from the neurosurgeon's point of view is evaluated.

Selection of Therapeutic Alternative

Safety

From the author's personal experiences, in 169 patients treated with GDC embolization, there were no mortality, 8 cases (4.7%) had permanent neurological deficits, while in the recent consecutive 80 cases treated with direct surgery, there were no mortality and 2.5% (2 cases) of morbidity. There is no significant difference between coil embolization and direct surgery as to the periprocedural mortality and morbidity.

Efficacy

As for efficacy of treatments, short term and long term efficacy of each treatment modality should be discussed separately.

In the series of 112 patients treated with GDC in the acute phase of SAH, acute subsequent bleeding occurred in only one case following GDC embolization. GDC embolization has been successful in preventing acute subsequent bleeding.

As for subarachnoid clot clearance, clot clearance in cases treated with GDC embolization is almost the same as that of direct surgery. Preservation of normal CSF pathway following GDC embolization might facilitate subarachnoid clot clearance.

As for symptomatic vasospasm, in the series of 112 patients treated with GDC in the acute phase of SAH, only 2 patients developed ischemic neurological deficits. In published series, the frequency and severity of vasospasm may be same in cases treated with GDC as in cases treated by direct surgery [1, 10]. It is one of the great advantage of coil embolization to occlude the aneurysm without manipulations of the brain parenchyma and the cerebral vasculatures. The frequency of hydrocephalus, like that of vasospasm, may be same in cases treated with GDC as in cases treated by direct surgery [9]. In summary, short term efficacy of coil embolization may be almost same as that of direct surgery.

In contrast to short term efficacy, long term efficacy of coil embolization is less satisfactory. In 169 patients treated with GDC embolization, there were 3 cases of delayed bleeding and 2 cases of thrombo-embolic events in cases treated with GDC. On follow up angiography, 13.5% of incompletely obliterated aneurysms exhibited progressive thrombosis, 21.6% remained unchanged and 64.9% displayed recanalization or regrowth on follow up angiography (Fig. 1).

Follow-up results are less satisfactory in cases involving incompletely obliterated lesions, whereas there is no doubt about long term durability of surgical clipping.

Figs. 3 and 4 demonstrate the representative case of delayed bleeding following GDC embolization. This 83 year-old lady had a left oculomotor palsy, and angiogram revealed IC-P-com aneurysm. Endovascular coil embolization resulted in incomplete occlusion and her oculomotor palsy once improved. Her oculomotor palsy recurred 1 year after the procedure, and angiogram demonstrated coil compaction and aneurysmal regrowth. She rejected further treatment. Two weeks after follow-up angiogram, she had severe subarachnoid hemorrhage.

long term angiographical follow up results

incomplete occlusion   37 cases

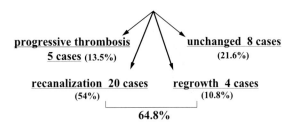

progressive thrombosis   unchanged 8 cases
5 cases (13.5%)   (21.6%)

recanalization 20 cases   regrowth 4 cases
(54%)   (10.8%)

64.8%

Fig. 1. Long-term angiographical follow up results of incompletely obliterated aneurysms following GDC embolization

Endovascular treatment for aged patient
WFNS grade & GOS (≥75y.o.)

GOS grade	GR	MD	SD	V	D
I	●●●● ●		●		
II	●●●● ●		●		
III	●				
IV	●●	●●	●●	●●●● ●●	●●
V				●	●

Fig. 2. Results of GDC embolization for patients with ages over 75 with acute SAH. About 90% of grade 1 to 3 patients had good recovery

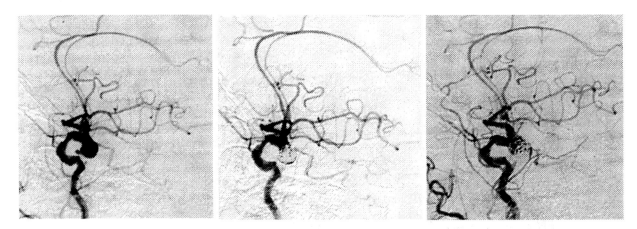

Fig. 3. 83 year-old lady with left oculomotor palsy. *Left:* Left carotid angiogram revealed IC-P-com aneurysm. *Center:* Left carotid angiogram obtained following endovascular coil embolization demonstrating incomplete occlusion of aneurysm. *Right:* Left carotid angiogram obtained 1 year after GDC embolization demonstrating coil compaction and aneurysmal regrowth

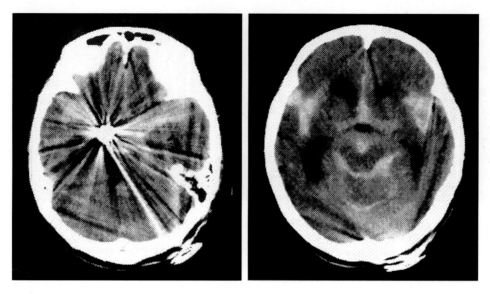

Fig. 4. A CT obtained 13 months after GDC embolization demonstrating severe SAH

A   **B**   **C**   **D**

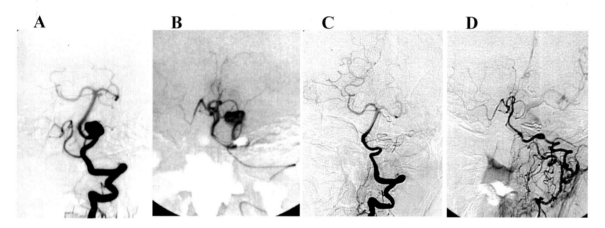

Fig. 5. 65 year-old lady with a ruptured left VA-PICA aneurysm. (A) Left vertebral angiogram demonstrating a VA-PICA aneurysm and a small BA-SCA aneurysm. (B) An aneurysmography via a micro-catheter introduced into the dome of aneurysm demonstrating the left PICA originating from neck of aneurysm. (C) Left vertebral angiogram obtained after clipping of the aneurysm demonstrating complete exclusion of the aneurysm from the circulation. (D) Left external carotid angiogram demonstrating a wide patency of OA-PICA anastomosis

Aneurysms with normal branching from their necks or domes and/or aneurysms with mass effects are also contraindication for GDC embolization. Such aneurysms could be treated by direct surgery with vascular reconstruction (Figs. 5, 6).

Degree of Invasion

As for the degree of invasion, coil embolization may be apparently less invasive than direct surgery, especially for aged patients and patients with poor medical conditions. Fig. 2 shows the results of GDC embolization for patients with ages over 75 with acute SAH. About 90% of grade 1 to 3 patients had good recovery.

Cost of Treatment

As for cost of treatment, coil embolization is almost same as direct surgery in cases with small aneurysm, while in large or giant aneurysm, direct surgery may be more cost effective than coil embolization.

In summary, the most important advantage of direct surgery is long term durability, while conditions of patients and aneurysmal geometry limit the indication of direct surgery. In contrast, the most serious disadvantage of coil embolization is long term durability, while medical condition of patients and aneurysmal geometry do not affect the indication of coil embolization.

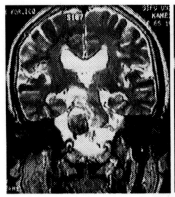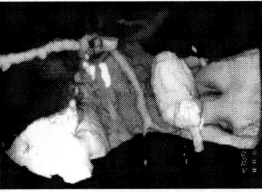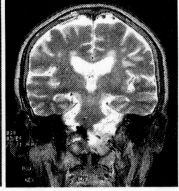

Fig. 6. *Left:* An MRI demonstrating a giant partially thrombosed right vertebral aneurysm with surrounding brain edema. *Center:* A 3D-CT angiogram demonstrating the precise configuration and location of aneurysm. *Right:* An MRI obtained after direct surgery, trapping of aneurysm and transposition of the PICA from the aneurysmal neck to the proximal vertebral artery and removal of intraluminal thrombus, demonstrating remarkable shrinkage of aneurysm and alleviation of mass effect

Discussion

Endovascular embolization using GDCs for complicated intracranial aneurysms has become widely accepted as an alternative to direct surgery. Published reports of early clinical and angiographical results have been promising [3], but the long term efficacy of the GDC methods remains to be undetermined. Incomplete endovascular occlusion of aneurysm leaves the patient at risk for future expansion and future subarachnoid hemorrhage [5, 7]. Hayakawa *et al.* evaluated the anatomical evolution of neck remnants in aneurysms treated with GDCs [4]. They reported that 25% of aneurysms with neck remnant exhibited progressive thrombosis, 26% remained unchanged and 49% displayed recanalization on follow up angiography. Especially in large or giant aneurysms, 88% of aneurysm with neck remnant displayed aneurysmal recanalization. As with their follow up results, 64.9% of incompletely obliterated aneurysms showed aneurysmal recanalization or regrowth in this series.

The size of an aneurysm neck correlates well with the initial morphological results of the endovascular treatment for cerebral aneurysms [11]. In the cases with wide-necked aneurysm, neointimal formation across the aneurysm neck was rarely completed, furthermore, looser packing with GDCs may prevent neointimal and neoendothelial proliferation across the neck of the aneurysm. Therefore, the coils and the unorganized intra-aneurysmal thrombus were directly exposed to the blood circulation. Subsequently, the coils can be pushed by the arterial pressure and become compacted toward the aneurysm dome with further expansion of the aneurysm.

With this limitation in mind, patients need to be very carefully chosen for GDC embolization and strict follow-up angiography is mandatory when a complete embolization is not achieved.

Conclusions

GDC embolization is a safe treatment with low incidence of periprocedural morbidity, and has been successful in preventing acute subsequent bleeding, whereas follow-up results are less satisfactory in cases involving incompletely obliterated lesions. High incidence of recanalization was promoted in cases with neck remnant and/or body filling. Further refinements of GDC technology is necessary to improve present morphological and clinical outcomes. As long term durability of endovascular aneurysm treatment is still less satisfactory, patients need to be very carefully chosen for GDC embolization.

References

1. Gruber A, Ungersböck K, Reinprecht A, Czech T, Gross C, Bednar M, Richling B (1988) Evaluation of cerebral vasospasm after early surgical and endovascular treatment of ruptured intracranial aneurysms. Neurosurgery 42: 258–268
2. Gruber DP, Zimmerman GA, Tomsick TA, van Loveren HR, Link MJ, Tew Jr JM (1999) A comparison between endovascular and surgical management of basilar artery apex aneurysms. J Neurosurg 90: 868–874
3. Guglielmi G, Viñuela F, Dion J, Duckwiler GR (1991) Electrothrombosis of saccular aneurysms via endovascular approach. Part 2: preliminary clinical experience. J Neurosurg 75: 8–14
4. Hayakawa M, Murayama Y, Duckwiler GR, Gobin YP, Guglielmi G, Viñuela F (2000) Natural history of the neck remnant of a cerebral aneurysm treated with the Guglielmi detachable coil system. J Neurosurg 93: 561–568

5. Hodgson TJ, Carroll T, Jellinek DA (1998) Subarachnoid hemorrhage due to late recurrence of a previously unruptured aneurysm after complete endovascular occlusion. AJNR 19: 1939–1941

6. Koivisto T, Vanninen R, Hurskainen H, Saari T, Hernesniemi J, Vapalahti M (2000) Outcomes of early endovascular versus surgical treatment of ruptured cerebral aneurysms. A prospective randomized study. Stroke 31: 2369–2377

7. Mericle RA, Wakhloo AK, Lopes DK, Lanzino G, Guterman LR, Hopkins LN (1998) Delayed aneurysm regrowth and recanalization after Guglielmi detachable coil treatment. J Neurosurg 89: 142–145

8. Regli L, Uske A, Tribolet N (1999) Endovascular coil placement compared with surgical clipping for the treatment of unruptured middle cerebral artery aneurysms: a consecutive series. J Neurosurg 90: 1025–1030

9. Sethi H, Moore A, Dervin J, Clifton A, MacSweeney JE (2000) Hydrocephalus: comparison of clipping and embolization in aneurysm treatment. J Neurosurg 92: 991–994

10. Yalamanchili K, Rosenwasser RH, Thomas JE, Liebman K, McMorrow C, Cannon P (1998) Frequency of cerebral vasospasm in patients treated with endovascular occlusion of intracranial aneurysms. AJNR 19: 553–558

11. Zubillaga AF, Guglielmi G, Viñuela F, Duckwiler GR (1994) Endovascular occlusion of intracranial aneurysms with electrically detachable coils: correlation of aneurysm neck size and treatment results. AJNR 15: 815–820

Correspondence: Yasuhiko Kaku, M.D., Department of Neurosurgery, Gifu University School of Medicine, 40 Tsukasamachi, Gifu 500-8705, Japan.

Acta Neurochir (2002) [Suppl] 82: 105–118

Strategies for Surgical Management of Cerebral Aneurysms of Special Location, Size and Form – Approach, Technique and Monitoring

Y. Yonekawa, N. Khan, and **P. Roth**

Department of Neurosurgery, University Hospital Zurich, Zurich, Switzerland

Summary

Special strategies are mandatory for optimal surgical management of aneurysms of special location, size and form. Approaches of extradural selective anterior clinoidectomy, partial occipital condylectomy, transpetrosal approach by anterior petrosectomy and supracerebellar transtentorial approach are discussed among them. Furthermore various types of temporary and permanent clipping procedures are discussed along with mention of intraoperative monitoring.

Keywords: Approach; temporary clipping; intraoperative monitoring; aneurysm surgery.

Introduction

Strategies applied for frequently encountered cerebral aneurysms in addition to our structured treatment have been discussed elsewhere [32] and also by other authors in this book. It is the aim of this paper to communicate our strategy of surgical management of aneurysms that are less frequent but are present in a special location and are of an abnormal size and form, making radical clipping difficult and problematic. Hunterian ligation with or without bypass procedure or other procedures such as coating of aneurysms are beyond the scope of this communication. Strategies of direct neck clipping surgery have to be changed according to angiographic anatomical findings of aneurysms concerned. This has been partly discussed elsewhere [34].

Approaches

Selection of surgical approaches is of cardinal importance in the management of aneurysms of special location and size. This is to be done in accordance with

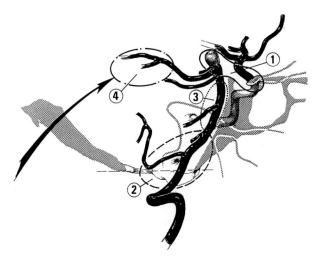

Fig. 1. Angiographical anatomical location of aneurysms and approaches. *1* SEAC, *2* Lateral suboccipital transcondylar approach, *3* Subtemporal transpetrosal approach, *4* SCTT approach

angio-anatomical findings of aneurysms (Fig. 1). Selective extradural anterior clinoidectomy covers special aneuryms of the anterior circulation especially of paraclinoid aneurysms along with aneurysms of the upper portion of the basilar artery with aneurysmal necks located above the level of the posterior clinoid process. Subtemporal approach with or without anterior petrosectomy covers anreurysms of the basilar artery with aneurysmal necks located below the level of the posterior clinoid process. The lateral suboccipital craniotomy frequently combined with a partial occipital condylectomy solves the problems of special aneurysms arising from the vertebral artery. The supracerebellar transtentorial approach enables us to reach distal parts of the posterior cerebral artery PCA.

*Selective Extradural Anterior Clinoidectomy SEAC:
(For the Management of Basilar Tip Aneuryms,
Basilar Superior Cerebellar BA-SCA Aneurysms,
Paraclinoid Aneurysms) (Fig. 2)*

Intradural removal of part of the anterior clinoid process for the management of some internal carotid artery aneurysms *i.e.* carotid-ophthalmic aneurysms was already performed at the end of the 1950's and reported in the 1970's and thereafter [18, 23, 30, 31]. Extensive extradural removal of the sphenoid ridge including orbital roof to manage such aneurysms was reported by Dolenc [7]. Modification of this procedure has been applied for posterior circulation aneurysm surgery by Day, Fukusima *et al.* [5, 6]. SEAC initiated in 1993 and reported in 1997, is referred to in our previous paper [35].

The advantages of this procedure are: 1) wider working space and 2) better illumination. Not only in the case of basilar aneurysms (Fig. 3) but also in the case of large paraclinoid aneurysms (Fig. 4) this wider space becomes very important, as the perforation of the lamina terminalis, for the purpose of slackness of the brain as mentioned later, is dangerous due to the usual extension of the aneurysm dome of this type underneath the lamina, thus hindering decompression by CSF drainage. Hence this is the only space available for the management of ruptured large paraclinoid aneurysms. Better illumination achieved through this procedure can not be overemphasized, as this enables better discrimination of the in-depth anatomical situation. Drilling away of the posterior clinoid process should be added to enable a temporary clipping procedure or to allow permanent neck clipping for the low-positioned basilar tip aneurysms. Importance of the subtemporal approach for such aneurysms developed by Drake at the end of 1950 [8] and described in final details by Drake, Peerless and Hernesniemi in 1996 [9] cannot be overemphasized.

The SEAC approach is performed as follows: Combined with conventional pterional approach after Yasargil with the drilling away of the sphenoid ridge to the extent of exposure of the most lateral corner of the superior orbital fissure [28, 29]. A branch of the middle meningeal artery namely the meningo-orbital artery passes here and anastomoses with the lacrimal artery with or without formation of the Hyrtl canal. Drilling away of the sphenoid ridge at this corner is extended medially until it crosses the line of the roof of the optic canal which is then drilled away including the optic

strut at the most proximal corner of the canal. Removal of the anterior clinoid process can be followed en bloc in about 30% of patients (mostly younger patients having less dural adhesion with bone), in the rest of the patients the anterior clinoid process has to be removed piece-meal or by further drilling. The procedure is usually associated with two remarkable incidents: 1) profuse bleeding from the venous system in the clinoid space (not necessarily from the cavernous sinus) and 2) frequently with arrythmia due to trigeminal irritation. The former can be managed by compression with hemostatic cellulose and sponge and slight elevation of the head by tilting the operating table and the latter by topical application of procaine. The anesthesiologist should be informed beforehand in order to respond accordingly.

Attention should be drawn to two serious complications of this procedure: 1) optic nerve injury and 2) CSF rhinorrhea. To prevent optic nerve injury, one has to master the microsurgical drilling technique by cadaver dissection prior to clinical application. As for the latter one has to know beforehand the risk of this problem at the time of evaluation of neuroimaging, namely extension of the sphenoid sinus into the clinoid process. Betadine® disinfection and sealing with muscle and glue combined with a spinal drainage for a couple of days usually suffice to solve the problem. Only one case out of around 100 cases underwent treatment of transnasal sinus tamponade of fatty tissue by ENT surgeon.

Another important point worth mentioning is the selection of either a usual extradural approach prior to opening the dura or of an approach after the dural opening and confirming the intradural situation of the aneurysm. The latter is done for C3 aneurysms and C2 superior wall aneurysms in combination with prior exposure of the internal carotid artery at the neck in order to be able to manage an accidental rupture of aneurysms during the drilling procedure of the clinoid [15].

*Lateral Suboccipital Transcondylar Approach: (for the
Management of Vertebral Artery VA Aneurysms
Including Vertebral Artery – Posterior Inferior
Cerebellar Artery VA–PICA Aneurysms, Distal PICA
Aneurysms and VA Union Aneurysms) (Fig. 5)*

Initially this approach was considered to be useful and effective to manage the VA–PICA aneurysms located near the foramen magnum [34] (Fig. 6), but this

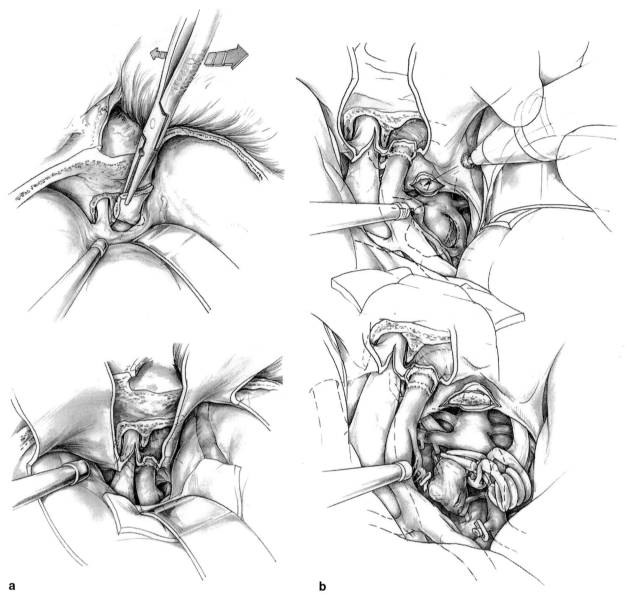

a   b

Fig. 2. Artist's drawing of SEAC (selective extradural anterior clinoidectomy) (a) a case with basilar tip aneurysm in which the posterior clinoid process is to be drilled away (b) and of a case with paraclinoid aneurysm (c)

has now turned out to be useful also for the above
mentioned aneurysms of every location.
The advantages are as follows:

– Excellent proximal control due to the possibility of
  putting a temporary clip to the extradural vertebral
  artery without touching the lower cranial nerves.
– Extensive view of the whole segment of the VA between the point just before the entrance into the
  dura and the vertebral union around the midline [3,
  13, 16]. This enables an appropriate placement of a
  temporary or permanent clip. If need be, vascular

reconstructive surgery can be performed with the
use of extradural segment of the vertebral artery.

The procedure is performed as follows:

1. Classical lateral suboccipital craniotomy by a linear
   incision in the retroauricular and retromastoid region.
2. Its enlargement until a part of the foramen magnum
   is opened and the medial part of the occipital condyle along with the condylar vein comes into sight.
   At this stage the horizontal segment of the vertebral

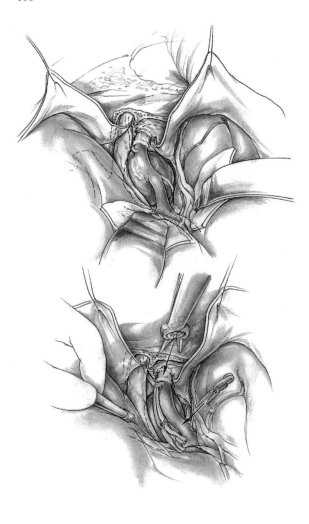

c

Fig. 2. (continued)

of the cerebellar tonsil and/or the biventer lobule, good exposure of the whole stretch of the intradural VA including the origin of the PICA and the VA union is achieved. At the time of dural incision, the accessory nerve should be paid attention to and not to be severed. At the very initial part of the intradural VA, the dentate ligament and the hypoglossal nerve come into sight.

5. The jugular tubercle is drilled away epidurally or intradurally, if needed, to get better access to the midline [21].

In this procedure the following points must be considered and avoided: 1) Air embolism in case of the sitting position (condylar vein, venous plexus around the VA, epidural and dural venous system at the craniocervical junction). 2) Injury of the VA at the time of extradural preparation. 3) Accessory nerve injury at the time of the dural incision.

Subtemporal Transpetrosal Approach with Anterior Petrosectomy: (for the Management of Basilar Trunk Aneurysms) (Fig. 7)

Basilar trunk aneurysms have been frequently managed using the subtemporal transtentorial approach [9]. Its combination with anterior petrosectomy [14] (drilling away of the bone posterior to the V3 root, medial to the greater petrosal nerve and anterior to the internal acoustic canal followed by transection of the superior petrosal sinus) enables better access to the basilar trunk located around the midline providing better illumination and wider working space as indicated in the SEAC procedure mentioned above.

Caution should be directed to prevent the following complications at the time of petrosectomy: 1) facial nerve palsy (greater petrosal nerve, facial nerve at the internal auditory canal), 2) hearing disturbance, 3) abducens palsy.

Figure 7 represents a case of ruptured basilar trunk aneurysm referred to us as an uncoilable case due to broadness of the neck.

Supracerebellar Transtentorial SCTT Approach: (for P2 and/or. P2–P3 Junction Aneurysms) (Fig. 8)

This approach enables access to the P2, P2/3 junction without retraction of the temporal lobe or without danger of compromising the vein of Labbé, especially important in the dominant hemisphere. Although details have been described elsewhere [33], outline of this

artery just before its dural entrance and also the nerve root C1 should come into sight.

3. The medial part of the occipital condyle is drilled away until the whole plane of the VA at the dural entrance is dissected, this makes a VA transposition feasible, if necessary. The condylar vein is frequently sacrificed at the time of the drilling. There is usually no need to drill away the corresponding condyle facet of the C1.

4. The dura is incised linearly just from the cranial part of the VA at its dural entrance towards the transverse sinus. Usually no additional incision is necessary. With this opening and slight retraction

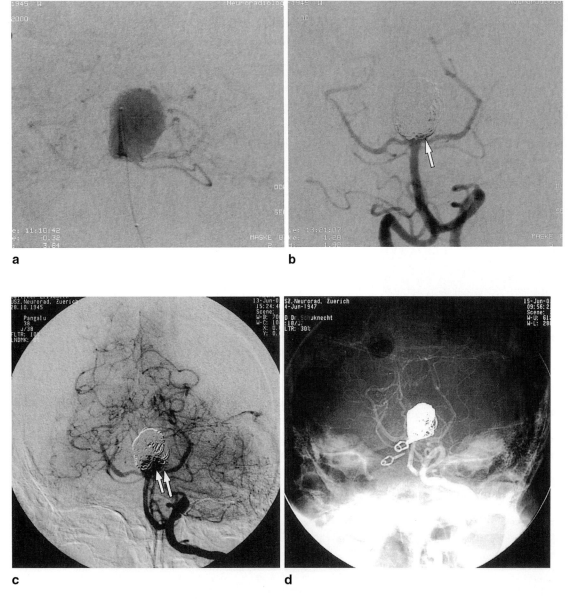

Fig. 3. A case of large basilar tip aneurysm (a) which was successfully coiled with some dog ear (↑) (b) but recanalized (↑↑) due to coil packing found on follow-up angiography one year later (c). This was clipped successfully (d) for which SEAC was combined with the usual pterional approach. A small unruptured aneurysm of the posterior communicating artery in the way was occluded after the clipping of the basilar aneurysm. The postoperative CT (e) shows that the anterior clinoid process was removed (↑)

approach is as follows: A linear incision is placed between the midline and the mastoid followed by exposure of the squama occipitalis. The transverse sinus should come into sight at the cranial corner of craniotomy. After having opened the dura, enough working space between the tentorium and the cranial surface of the cerebellum can be obtained in the sitting position, along with effective measures like CSF

drainage by opening the cisterna magna and the sacrifice of some bridging veins between the tentorial veins or the transverse sinus and the cerebellum. After having cut about 2/3 of the tentorium at the medial part, the PCA (P2 and P2/P3 junction) is inspected so that aneurysms of this location can be managed without retraction of the temporal lobe or compromising its venous drainage.

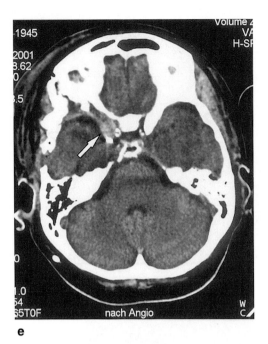

e

Fig. 3. (continued)

form, further tactics such as achievement of brain slackness, dissection of aneurysms, accomplishment of an ideal clipping are to be discussed.

Slackness of the Brain

Slackness of the brain namely to overcome the "angry brain" is mandatory for successful surgery in the acute stage of SAH

For this purpose, following measures are undertaken: 1) Administration of dehydrators such as mannitol. 2) Opening of the arachnoid membrane especially overlying the Sylvian fissure, and the basal cisterns, just after the dural opening. 3) Ventricular drainage 4) Opening of the Liliequist membrane 5) Opening of the lamina terminalis (ICA-, MCA-, AcomA, distal BA aneurysms) 6) Opening of the lateral ventricle by callosotomy (distal ACA aneurysms). 7) Opening of the cisterna cerebellomedularis (VA aneurysms).

Administration of mannitol is directed to its use as a protective agent against ischemia [36] rather than to reduce the swelling of the angry brain. Ventricular drainage is not routinely performed for the purpose to obtain slackness of the brain in cases with good clinical grading. Perforation of the lamina terminalis or transcallosal ventricular opening without ventricular drain-

Special Techniques

For the management and achievement of good surgical results of aneurysms of special location, size and

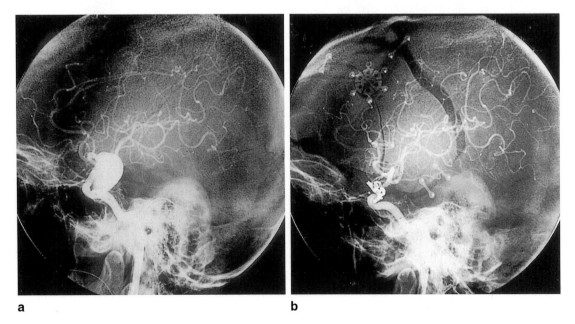

a   **b**

Fig. 4. A case of giant paraclinoid aneurysm: a: lateral view of preoperative b: postoperative angiography. Note the enlarged craniotomy. The bone flap was removed primarily due to a massive swelling and replaced later, prior to this angiography

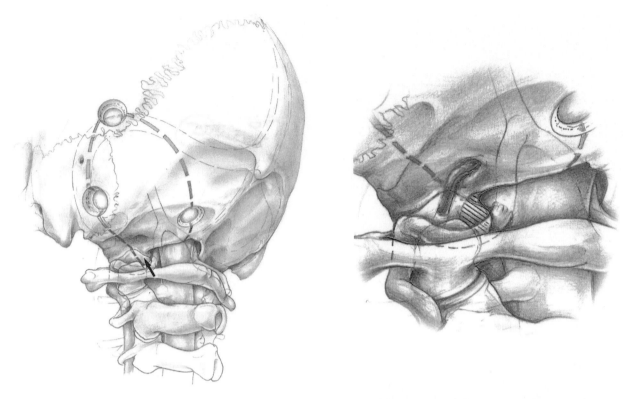

Fig. 5. Lateral suboccipital craniotomy combined with partial condylectomy. Note the condylectomy is limited only to dissect the entire entry part of the vertebral artery into the dura, so that the condylar facet of the C1 and/or the condylar vein may remain preserved

age are our routine procedure. The ventricular drainage is aimed at ICP-monitoring and treatment of raised intracranial pressure ICP in cases with poor clinical grading. Our strategy is completing craniotomy without any drainage [32], when possible, in order to preserve or to expand the normal subarachnoid space by letting the CSF irrigate the hemorrhagic space.

Clot Removal

Removal of the clot around a ruptured aneurysm and its neighbouring vessels has been reported to be of cardinal importance to prevent vasospasm [27]. On the other hand excessive vascular manipulation during surgical procedure is considered to be harmful for fear of induction of mechanical vasospasm. This point is especially important in the management of aneurysms of arteries harboring perforating arteries considered to be "end artery". Our strategy is to limit the clot removal around the ruptured aneurysm and its neighbouring arteries followed by topical application of papaverin [32].

Temporary Clipping, Temporary Trapping

Temporary clipping is an accepted procedure [36] used routinely for an ideal aneurysm neck clipping. Its advantages are as follows: 1) prevention and management of premature rupture at the time of aneurysm dissection. 2) slackness of aneurysms enables ideal neck clipping. The time-limitation allowed for temporary occlusion reported to date varies considerably [1, 32, 36]. Duration of 10–15 minutes has been reported to be acceptable. Temporary occlusion of the extracranial carotid artery or vertebral artery can be appropriate measure to manage paraclinoid internal carotid artery aneurysms or vertebral artery aneurysms.

Our strategy of temporary clipping is as follows: 1) administration of mannitol (20 gm i.v.) prior to temporary occlusion 2) duration of temporary occlusion to be limited to within 15 min 3) administration of barbiturates (thiopental 500 mg i.v.) when this duration exceeds 15 min 4) administration of heparin 2500 i.v. to prevent intravascular clot formation at the site of the temporary clip, when the time duration should exceed 30 min.

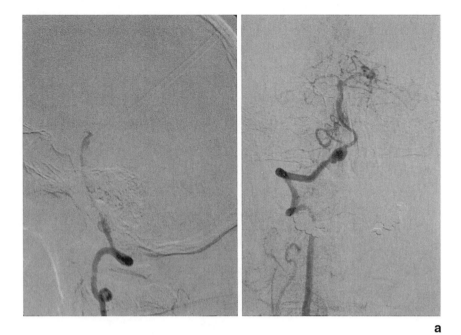

a

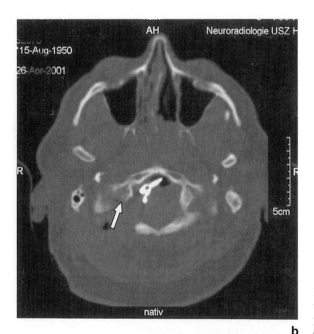

b

Fig. 6. A case of dissection aneurysm of the vertebral artery located near the midline and the foramen magnum (a). The aneurysm was trapped proximal to the posterior inferior cerebellar artery. Note the partial condylectomy (↑) on the postoperative CT scan (b)

The following points are to be considered for the application of a temporary clip: 1) Duration of the temporary clipping should be as short as possible in the case of remarkable brain swelling or intracerebral hematoma, where the surrounding microcirculation is always compromised. 2) Site of placement of clip at the concerned parent artery where some athromatous plaque is visible and remarkable should be avoided. 3)

Closing pressure of the temporary clip should be optimal to close the vessel but not to injure its wall and endothelium irreversibly. 4) Head(s) of temporary clip(s) should not interfere with the procedure of permanent clipping.

Temporary trapping is another special strategy of our aneurysm surgery especially for large and giant aneurysms. This enables bloodless puncturing of such

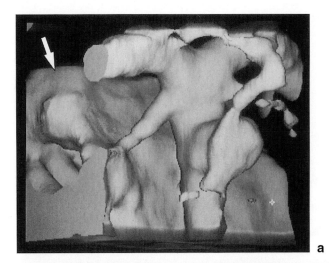

Fig. 7. A case of aneurysm of the basilar trunk: (a) preoperative 3D CT angiography showing that the aneurysm having a broad neck is directed to the pons and located lower to the level of the posterior clinoid process (↑). (b) postoperative angiography displayed a successful clipping of the aneurysm. (c) Postoperative CT scan showing direction of clip-insertion through the level of petrosectomy. A small clip is for the occlusion of the superior petrosal sinus

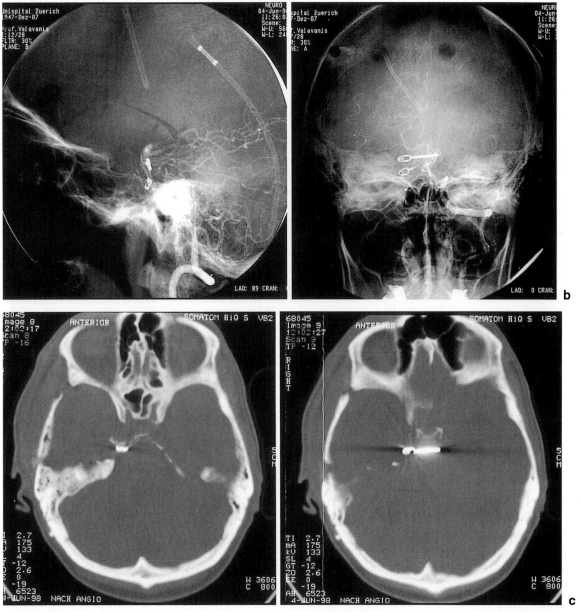

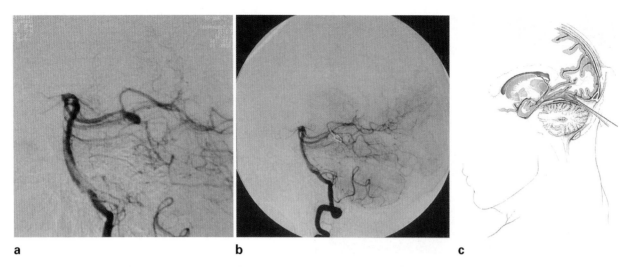

Fig. 8. A case of P2–P3 junction aneurysm: a. preoperative angiography. b. postoperative angiography showing successful clipping and c. artist's drawing of the SCTT approach

aneurysms ("puncture and collapse" method as mentioned later) so that perforators around the neck can be checked prior to placement of a permanent clip (Fig. 9). Optimal permanent clip(s) of form and size can be selected corresponding to the aneurysmal neck-parent artery relationship. The idea derives from the fact that the situation of cerebral blood flow (CBF) distal to the distal clips must be the same as that of the proximal temporary clip except for the perfusion territory of the trapped segment. Duration of temporary trapping, in which the "end arteries" such as the anterior choroidal artery and other perforating arteries like thalamo-perforating artery are included, should be therefore as short as possible in order to prevent their ischemic complications. Combination of hypothermia for safer temporary clipping procedure in the treatment of aneurysms concerned is another topic to be discussed separately in details [24, 25].

Clipping of Aneurysms

At the time of final clipping of an aneurysm, puncture of its dome and confirmation of its collapse is our routine procedure in order to check the completeness of the clipping and to examine the situation of the posterior side of clipped aneurysms (perforators, neck remnant, cranial nerves). This procedure would obviate use of endoscopic confirmation for this purpose [10, 22].

We therefore follow the below mentioned important techniques at the time of final clipping:

1) "puncture and collapse" method for the management of aneurysms combined with above mentioned temporary trapping obviates the complicated method of combining with intraoperative endovascular procedure for aneurysms of special location and size [17] (Fig. 10) and also obviates unnecessary use of multiple clips and clips of special forms. This method enables application of optimal clip(s) corresponding with the aneurysm neck-parent artery relationship.
2) Combination of fenestrated clip and standard clip as shown in Fig. 11 enables preservation of important vessels branching from the aneurysm neck or from the aneurysm dome as well as nerves passing near the aneurysm neck.
3) Double clipping: Large sized aneurysms have frequently atheromatous or calcified wall in the vicinity of the neck so that only one clip cannot close the lumen completely. Another clip just distal to the original clip would suffice for a complete occlusion.

Intraoperative Monitoring

It is our experience that an apparent complete clipping from a microsurgical view does not necessarily indicate completeness of the clipping. Blood flow

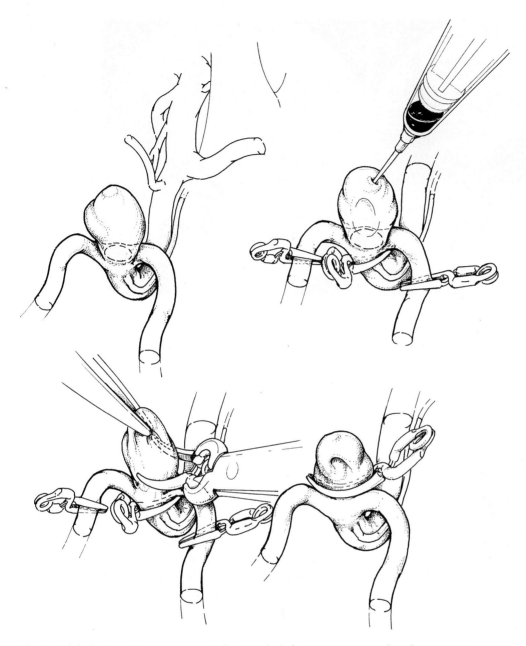

Fig. 9. Artist's drawing of the puncture and collapse method after a temporary trapping of an aneurysm

monitoring and neurophysiological monitoring are mandatory for this purpose: 1) MicroDoppler sonography: This is an important tool to check the patency of important vessels after an aneurysm clipping. Lack of blood flow quantification remains a disadvantage of this method but the handiness and reliability are of great clinical advantage [2, 12]. 2) Peltier stack: this apparatus of CBF measurement of thermal clearance reflects a real time change of CBF after the application of temporary clip and its restoration after removal of the clip and is useful especially in the management of aneurysms of the ICA and MCA territory [4, 19]. The quantitative nature of this measurement supplies useful information in the management of vascular reconstructive procedure when necessary. 3) Intraoperative ultrasound imaging: This is very useful to detect and locate some aneurysms placed distally or peripherally such as mycotic aneurysms or distal MCA aneurysms

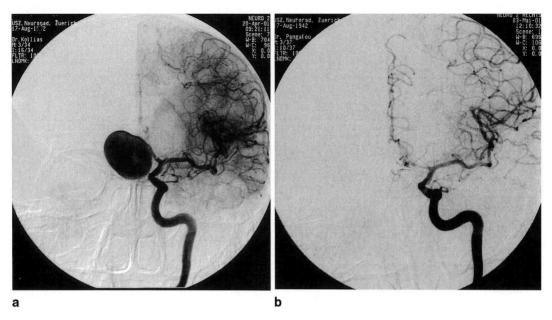

a   b

Fig. 10. A case of giant aneurysm of the anterior communicating artery presented with visual disturbance was successfully clipped with the mentioned "puncture and collapse" method. a. preoperative angiography. b. postoperative angiography

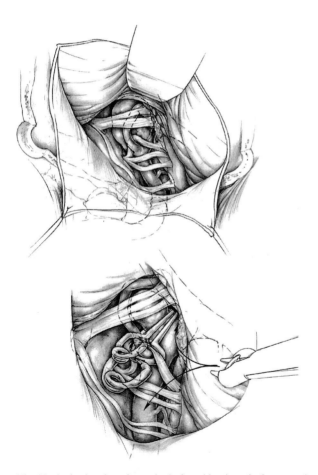

which are usually hidden deep in sulci and fissures [20]. 4) SEP: Restoration of neuronal function by releasing a temporary clip or by releasing a small perforator from an entanglement at the time of neck clipping can be registered by SEP monitoring [11, 26] (Fig. 12).

Conclusion

Our strategies of surgical management of intracranial aneurysms of special location, size and form are presented with detailed mention of the applied surgical approaches and techniques and intracranial monitoring necessary for optimal neck clipping. Selection of appropriate strategies and continuous refinement of surgical technique are mandatory for improvement of the clinical results of aneurysm surgery.

Acknowledgment

Authors are indebted to Ms. R. Frick for the secretarial assistance.

Fig. 11. Artist drawing of a method of combination of a fenestrated clip with a usual straight clip enabling preservation of the nerve and the PICA which is located at the neck of the aneurysm

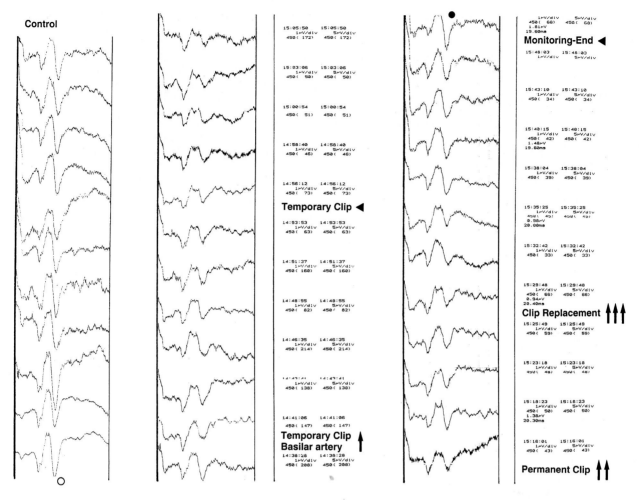

Fig. 12. Continuous SEP monitoring indicating abnormal SEP at the time of temporary clipping of the basilar artery (↑) and normalization after removal of the temporary clipping (↑↑) and also after releasing a perforating artery (↑↑↑) which was entangled at the site of neck clipping of a basilar trunk aneurysm. ○ beginning, ● end

References

1. Araki Y, Anroh H, Yamada M, Nakatani K, Andoh T, Sakai N (1999) Permissible arterial occlusion time in aneurysm surgery: Postoperative hyperperfusion caused by temporary clipping. Neuro Med Chir (Tokyo) 39: 901–907
2. Bailes JE, Tantuwaya LS, Fukushima T, Schurman GW, Davis D (1997) Intraoperative microvascular Doppler sonography in aneurysm surgery. Neurosurgery 40: 965–972
3. Bertalanffy H, Seeger W (1991) The dorsolateral suboccipital transcondylar approach to the lower clivus and anterior portion of the craniocervical junction. Neurosurgery 29: 815–821
4. Carter LP, White WL, Atkinson JR (1978) Regional cortical blood flow at craniotomy. Neurosurgery 2: 223–229
5. Day JD, Fukushima T, Giannotta SL (1997) Cranial base approaches to posterior circulation aneurysms. J Neurosurg 87: 544–554
6. Day JD, Giannota SL, Fukushima T (1994) Extradural temporopolar approach to lesions of the upper basilar artery and infrachiasmatic region. J Neurosurg 81: 230–235
7. Dolenc VV (1985) A combined epi- and subdural direct approach to carotid-ophthalmic artery aneurysms. J Neurosurg 62: 667–672
8. Drake CG (1961) Bleeding aneurysms of the basilar artery. Direct surgical management in four cases. J Neurosurg 18: 230–238
9. Drake CG, Peerless S, Hernesniemi J (1996) The subtemporal approach. In: Drake CG, Peerless S, Hernesniemi J (eds) Surgery of vertebrobasilar aneurysms. Springer, Wien New York, pp 21–26
10. Fischer J, Mustafa H (1994) Endoscopic-guided clipping of cerebral aneurysms. Br J Neurosurg 8: 559–565
11. Friedman WA, Kaplan BL, Day AL, Sypert GW, Curran MT (1987) Evoked potential monitoring during aneurysm operation: Observation after fifty cases. Neurosurgery 20: 678–687
12. Gilsbach JM (1984) Intraoperative Dopplersonography in Neurosurgery. Springer, Wien New York, pp 104
13. Kawase T, Bertalanffy H, Shiobara R, Otani M, Toya S, Shinozaki T, Ibata Y (1993) Difference of surgical field between the lateral suboccipital approach and the transcondylar approach for the midline vertebral aneurysms. Surg Cereb Stroke (Jpn) 21: 263–268
14. Kawase T, Toya S, Shiobara R, Mine T (1985) Transpetrosal approach for aneurysms of the lower basilar artery. J Neurosurg 63: 857–861
15. Korosue H, Heros RC (1992) "Subclinoid" carotid aneurysm

with erosion of the anterior clinoid process and fatal intra-oprative rupture. Neurosurgery 31: 356–360

16. Matsushima T, Fukui M (1996) Lateral approaches to the foramen magnum: With special reference to the transcondylar fossa approach and transcondylar approach. No Shinkei Geka 24: 119–124

17. Mizoi K, Takahashi A, Yoshimoto T, Fujiwara S, Koshu K (1993) Combined endovascular and neurosurgical approach for paraclinoid internal carotid artery aneurysms. Neurosurgery 33: 986–992

18. Morgan F (1972) Removal of anterior clinoid process in the surgery of carotid aneurysm, with some notes on recurrent subarachnoid hemorrhage during craniotomy. Schweiz Arch Neurol Neurochir Psychiatr 111: 363–368

19. Ogata N, Fournier Y, Imhof HG, Yonekawa Y (1996) Thermal diffusion blood flow monitoring during aneurysm surgery. Acta Neurochir (Wien) 138: 726–731

20. Payer M, Kaku Y, Bernays R, Yonekawa Y (1998) Intraoperative color-coded duplex sonography for localization of a distal middle cerebral artery aneurysm: Technical case report. Neurosurgery 42: 941–943

21. Perneczky A (1986) The posterolateral approach to the foramen magnum. In: Samii M (ed) Surgery in and around the brain stem and the third ventricle. Springer, Berlin Heidelberg New York Tokyo, pp 460–466

22. Perneczky A, Fries G (1998) Endoscope assisted brain surgery: part 1. Evolution, basic concept, and current technique. Neurosurgery 42: 219–225

23. Perneczky A, Knosp E, Vorkapic P, Czech T (1985) Direct surgical approach to infraclinoidal aneurysms. Acta Neurochir (Wien) 76: 36–44

24. Satoh A, Nakamura H, Kobayashi S, Kageyama Y, Miyata A, Kadoh K, Nakamura T, Itoh N, Wtanabe Y (1999) Usefulness of hypothermic anesthesia in surgery for cerebral aneurysm. Surg Cerb Stroke (Jpn) 27: 183–188

25. Spetzler RF, Hadley MN, Rigamonti D, Carter LP, Raudzens PA, Shedd SA, Wilkinson E (1988) Aneurysms of the basilar artery treated with circulatory arrest hypothermia, and barbiturate cerebral protection. J Neurosurg 68: 868–879

26. Symon L, Wang AD, Costa e Silva IE, Gentili F (1984) Perioperative use of somatosensory evoked responses in aneurysm surgery. J Neurosurg 60: 269–275

27. Taneda M (1982) Effect of early operation for ruptured aneurysms on prevention of delayed ischemic symptoms. J Neurosurg 57: 622–628

28. Yasargil MG, Antic J, Laciga R, Jain KK, Hodosh RM, Smith RD (1976) Microneurosurgical pterional approach to aneurysms of the basilar bifurcation. Surg Neurol 6: 83–91

29. Yasargil MG, Fox JL, Ray MW (1975) The operative approach to aneurysms of the anterior communicating artery. Adv Tech Stand Neurosurg 2: 113–170

30. Yasargil MG, Gasser JC, Hodosh RM, Rankin TV (1977) Carotid-ophthalmic aneurysms: Direct microsurgical approach. Surg Neurol 8: 155–165

31. Yasargil MG (1984) Carotid-posterior communicating aneurysms. Chapter 2. Internal carodit artery aneurysms. In: Yasargil MG (ed) Microneurosurgery. Clinical coniderations, surgery of the intercranial aneurysms and results, vol II. Thieme, Stuttgart, pp 78–81

32. Yonekawa Y, Imhof HG, Ogata N, Bernays R, Kaku Y, Fandino J, Taub E (1998) Aneurysm surgery in the acute stage: Results of structured treatment. Neurol Med Chir (Tokyo) [Suppl] 38: 45–49

33. Yonekawa Y, Imhof HG, Taub E, Curcic M, Kaku Y, Roth P, Wieser HG, Groscurth P (2001) Supracerebellar transtentorial approach to posterior temporomedial structures. J Neurosurg 94: 339–345

34. Yonekawa Y, Kaku Y, Imhof HG, Kiss M, Curcic M, Taub E, Roth P (1999) Posterior circulation aneurysms. Technical strategies based on angiographic anatomical findings and the results of 60 recent consecutive cases. Acta Neurochir (Wien) [Suppl] 72: 123–140

35. Yonekawa Y, Ogata N, Imhof HG, Olivecrona M, Strommer K, Kwak TE, Roth P, Groscurth P (1997) Selective extradural anterior clinoidectomy for supra- and parasellar processes. Technical note. J Neurosurg 87: 636–642

36. Yoshimoto T, Suzuki J (1976) Intracranial definitive aneurysm surgery under normothermia and normotension-utilizing temporary occlusion of major cerebral arteries and preoperative mannitol administration. No Shinkei Geka 4: 775–783 (Jpn, with Eng abstract)

Correspondence: Y. Yonekawa, Department of Neurosurgery, University Hospital, Frauenklinik Str. 10, 8091 Zurich, Switzerland.

Author Index

Index of Keywords

SpringerMedicine

Hans-Jakob Steiger et al.

Neurosurgery of Arteriovenous Malformations and Fistulas

A Multimodal Approach

2002. VIII, 473 pages. 617 figures, partly in colour.
Hardcover **EUR 228,–**
(Recommended retail price) Net-prices subject to local VAT.
ISBN 3-211-83703-5

Arteriovenous malformations (AVM) and fistulas (AVF) differ from all other pathology affecting the central nervous system by their high-flow arteriovenous shunts. Permanent occlusion of these shunts is the essence and the challenge of therapy. Much progress has been made since the first neurosurgical efforts to deal with these problems. Endovascular therapy and radiosurgery became accepted alternatives or adjuncts to surgery. In many instances the choice of the primary therapeutic modality is not clear and arguments can be found for several options. However, microsurgery, endovascular therapy and radiosurgery differ very much with regard to invasiveness, length of stay at the hospital but also residual risk after therapy. These secondary factors are often decisive for the choice of treatment modality. The book presents in a clearly structured way the modern treatment concepts. It has been written for all colleagues involved in surgery, radiosurgery and endovascular therapy of neurovascular malformations.

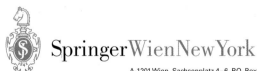

SpringerWienNewYork

A-1201 Wien, Sachsenplatz 4–6, P.O. Box 89, Fax +43.1.330 24 26, e-mail: books@springer.at, Internet: **www.springer.at**
D-69126 Heidelberg, Haberstraße 7, Fax +49.6221.345-229, e-mail: orders@springer.de
USA, Secaucus, NJ 07096-2485, P.O. Box 2485, Fax +1.201.348-4505, e-mail: orders@springer-ny.com
Eastern Book Service, Japan, Tokyo 113, 3–13, Hongo 3-chome, Bunkyo-ku, Fax +81.3.38 18 08 64, e-mail: orders@svt-ebs.co.jp